"Nicole Bell's book, *What Lurks in the Woods*, is a personal journey; raw, real, and heartfelt. If we all knew what Nicole describes in her book, Alzheimer's could be a much less common disease. For anyone with a family member with cognitive decline or risk for decline, this book provides a kindred spirit of support and knowledge. I recommend it highly."

—**Dr. Dale Bredesen, MD**, Professor,
Author of the *New York Times* bestseller *The End of Alzheimer's*

"This book is a private window into the pain and destruction caused by chronic illness. Nicole Bell's passion for finding the root cause of her husband's illness is awe-inspiring, and those suffering from medical mysteries will learn much from her journey. *What Lurks in the Woods* is a powerful story that will reframe your view of modern medicine."

—**Dana Parish**, co-author of the best-selling book, *Chronic,*
Sony Music singer/songwriter

"*What Lurks in the Woods* is a raw and wrenching memoir that will jolt you out of the fairy tale that doctors have it all figured out. Spoiler alert—we don't. But real answers start with the right questions, and Nicole Bell asks them in abundance. May her tragic journey of discovery help others to find their way."

—**Dr. Steven Phillips, MD,**
Co-author of the best-selling book, *Chronic*

"In this courageous memoir, Nicole Bell describes her beloved husband's descent into early dementia and the cruel realization that his disease was fueled by a mix of undiagnosed tick-borne diseases. This riveting narrative is a must-read for caregivers of mentally ill loved ones who are searching for answers in the face of a medical system unwilling to seriously explore the links between microbes and mental illness."

—**Kris Newby**, science writer,
Author of *BITTEN: The Secret History of Lyme Disease and Biological Weapons*

"*What Lurks in the Woods* is a powerful example of a real-life hardship caused by the trials and travels of tick-borne illness. Nicole Bell artfully captures the painful emotions, confusion, and heartache that permeate patients and their families. The story is captivating, and the vivid detail brought me into the room through every twist and turn. Bell also highlights the incompleteness of traditional medical treatment and encourages those on a similar journey to reject the typical rhetoric that there is no hope. Anyone dealing with chronic illness will connect with this book."

—Dr. Chris Turnpaugh, MD,
President and Founder of Turnpaugh Health and Wellness Center

"*What Lurks in the Woods* is a captivating story of one family's struggle to make sense of a heart-breaking diagnosis of early-onset Alzheimer's disease and the potential role that subclinical infections could have played in the irreversible damage caused over more than a decade. It is a must-read for those investigating the role of infection in chronic disease, including researchers and advocates in the Alzheimer's disease and tickborne disease communities. I couldn't put it down!"

—Dr. Amanda Elam,
CEO and Co-founder of Galaxy Diagnostics, Inc.

"This is a heart-wrenching love story and intimate memoir of profound loss at the cruel hands of Alzheimer's Disease. Impeccably detailed, this is a wife's journey navigating a complex medical landscape, leveraging her brilliant scientific mind to unveil the origin of her husband's Alzheimer's. *What Lurks in the Woods* calls attention to decades of research suggesting that infectious, immune, and lifestyle factors are all important in the development of this horrific disease. It is a poignant call-to-action for the medical and research communities to develop precise, early strategies for assessing and treating Alzheimer's patients."

—Nikki Shultek,
Principal and Founder of Intracell Research Group

WHAT LURKS
IN THE WOODS

WHAT LURKS IN THE WOODS

STRUGGLE AND HOPE IN THE MIDST OF CHRONIC ILLNESS

A Memoir

NICOLE BELL

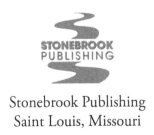

Stonebrook Publishing
Saint Louis, Missouri

A STONEBROOK PUBLISHING BOOK

Library of Congress Control Number: 2021910937

Paperback ISBN: 978-1-955711-01-2
eBook ISBN: 978-1-955711-02-9

www.stonebrookpublishing.net
PRINTED IN THE UNITED STATES OF AMERICA

For Ryan and Hailey

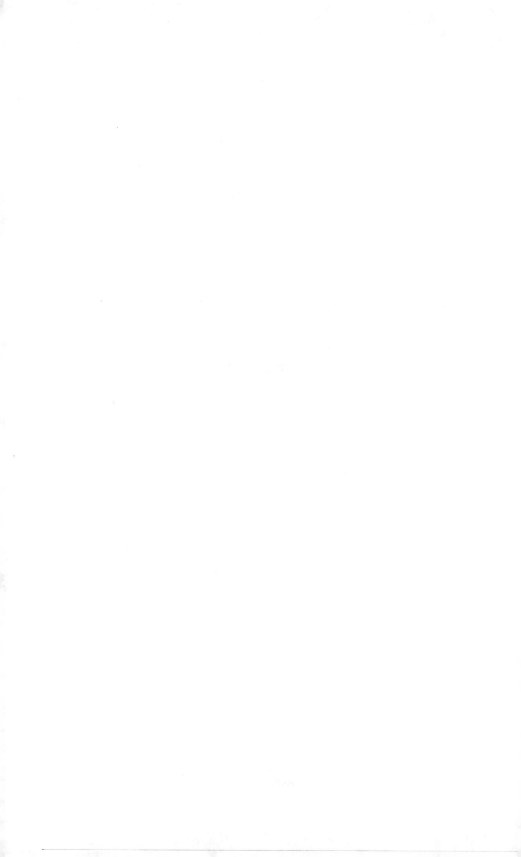

Contents

Introduction

I've always enjoyed writing. Even as a little girl, I overanalyzed the world around me. Conversations and events lingered and looped in my brain as if one more spin would unlock a hidden pattern. Life never provided the order and rules that I sought, but writing helped me discern which truths to hold on to and which to discard.

My high school English teacher once told me that I had a knack for creative fiction. It was a passing conversation more years ago than I care to admit, but it stuck with me because I knew he was wrong. Most of my writing wasn't fiction. The stories that received a coveted "8" on a scale of 1–5 came from actual events that my eager, pubescent mind struggled to digest. I changed some of the names and took minor liberties along the way, but it was pretty much life as it happened. The quirks and reflections of a middle-class, high school kid with a bit of my snark mixed in. Not Pulitzer Prize-winning, but heartfelt and real.

Eventually, the order and rules that I craved pulled me away from writing and toward engineering. Science and math had formulas and laws that described the world around me. One lecture unlocked the answers to thousands of problems, leaving an exponential impact. I was fascinated. After high school, MIT accepted me into their undergraduate program, and my life as an engineer began.

Years later, my slice of the world seemed perfect. My career thrived in a fast-paced, growing med-tech company, the smartest man I'd ever met was my best friend and husband, and I was a mom to two tiny humans who learned new things and amazed me every day. But piece by piece, that perfection crumbled, unearthing a harsh reality. My husband was sick. I followed the rules and paths laid out for me, but they led to more confusion. Root causes were a doctrine in engineering but were elusive in medicine. Without them, my husband sank deeper into his chronic illness.

Once again, thoughts circled, but this time the loops seemed infinite. They hovered over me throughout the night, preventing the rest that made sense of even a simple day. I wish I could say that I returned to writing as a thoughtful decision, but the reality was more desperate. One morning, the pounding treadmill in my head drowned out other rational thoughts. I opened my laptop to see if the loop preferred to run on the page. As it turned out, it did. Day after day, I typed, scribbled, and recorded audio when the words were too hard to face in print. Frantic journal entries poured out of me and helped me cope with the chaos.

Storms eventually pass, but once mine did, I still felt broken. Writing helped me escape the loops but didn't provide answers. Illness destroyed truths that I held dear, and only fragments and pieces remained in their place. I felt compelled to sort through the mess, process our journey, and discern what new truths had revealed themselves.

After a lot of thought, I decided to turn my journal entries into a book. At first, it felt like a project for me and those I loved. That would be enough. But the more I wrote, the more I processed, the more I distilled, I realized that wasn't enough. I wanted people who suffered from chronic illness to see my mistakes and successes and learn from them. I wanted them to trust their gut and realize that they're not alone. And if our story could help them see the signs, or ask the right questions, or find their root causes and answers *sooner*—well, maybe it would all be worth it.

So, Mr. Schauble, I guess I did write again. But, between you and me, I truly wish it had been fiction.

1

Telling Ryan

July 2017

"What the fuck are you doing?" For a moment, I thought this would be the last thing I ever said to my husband.

Russ took off right after I got home from work. Our friend, Susan, was there helping with the kids. She'd been a teacher at Ryan's daycare, and Russ and I fell in love with her energy and how she interacted with our son. However, recently, Russ said she was too loud and avoided her. He was also pissed because I asked him to stay at the house all morning to sign for a delivery that never came. Small stuff, but small stuff now sent him over the edge.

He went out for dinner. The GPS locator I put on his phone revealed his location—Tyler's Taproom. I groaned. I cooked low glycemic meals three times a day, and then he took off and ate a burger and fries when he got mad. Of course, he also drank. Alcohol made him lose his ability to compensate, so who knew what mess he would create when he got home.

At dinner, Ryan asked where Daddy was. I told him he went out. Usually, Ryan accepted that and moved on to another topic, but tonight, he mumbled something.

"What was that, babe?" I asked.

He mustered the confidence to speak. "I said, I know why he went out."

"You do? Why do you think that is?"

"Really? Do you want me to say it in front of Hailey?" Hailey looked up because she heard her name, but I could tell the conversation didn't engage her.

Now I was curious. "Yes, babe. What are you thinking?"

"I think he went out because he's disappointed in us."

The look on his face wrenched my gut like a wet rag. My sweet, emotional, seven-year-old boy thought he'd done something wrong. The words lingered—a glaring reminder of my inability to shelter him from the coming madness.

I hadn't told Ryan the whole truth. I'd skirted around the edges but never tackled it head-on. And my boy, who asked a zillion questions about everything, never asked. He noticed and watched and wanted to understand every little detail about everything, except this thing that mattered the most. A curious defense mechanism that I recognized but didn't hurry to combat. *Let him be a normal little boy a little longer. Let him idolize his dad for one more day or one more week.*

I knew it was time, but I didn't know how to have the conversation. How could I? How could I tell a little boy that he'd never know his real dad? The man I loved. The man who solved any problem, talked to any stranger, and made everyone laugh. How could I tell him that father-son events would be awkward and painful? That Mom would do her best to compensate but would never fill the void, and the life I envisioned for him would never happen? How could I tell him all that? On the other hand, how could I let his comment go unaddressed?

So, I told him—not the whole truth, but something a little deeper around the edges. Enough to understand that Dad wasn't healthy. That he did things that didn't seem to make sense or didn't seem fair. And when he did these things, it was okay to be upset, but it wasn't okay to turn that anger on his sister or me. We had to stick together, help each other, and help Dad because this problem wasn't his fault. He used to be able to control his anger, but he wasn't very good at that anymore.

"Will it get better? Can we help him get less angry?" Ryan asked. Another gut wrench.

"Well, sometimes Mommy can calm him down. I've gotten pretty good at that. But it takes time, and sometimes, the best thing to do is give him some space."

Ryan asked more questions, and I did my best to answer them. I tried not to go too far, and I tried not to scare him. When I felt like I'd told enough of the story, I asked, "Do you want to talk about it anymore? Do you have any questions?"

"No. I understand. I'm good."

Later that night, he asked how old he would have to be before I told him how babies were made. He also asked—six times—if I paid Susan to take care of him and Hailey in the afternoons. But no more questions about Dad.

Russ came home after I put the kids to bed, but he didn't come inside. I was too crabby and tired to care, so I ignored it and watched *American Horror Story*. It wasn't the best show for my mental well-being, but at least that alternate reality felt worse than mine.

Before going to bed, I made my rounds to lock up the house. In the garage, Russ stared at the darkness of an open door.

"What the fuck are you doing?" I asked.

Honestly, I didn't understand his answer. He mumbled something about the TV. Every ounce of me was exhausted, so I left him in the garage and went to bed. There was only so much one person could take.

The next morning, I found that Russ had never come to bed. He often slept in the living room or the guest bedroom when he got angry—even before. I checked my phone and saw a notification that he'd left the house at 5:50 a.m. He never left the house that early. The GPS showed that he was in the neighborhood. *Is he out for a walk? A bike ride?*

A big "R" denoted his location on my screen and was moving too slowly to indicate a bike ride. The dogs slept at their posts in the living room; he usually took them when he went for a walk. *What is he doing?*

I continued my morning routine, and still no Russ. Frustrated, I grabbed my phone and saw the "R" on an undeveloped lot in the neighborhood. *Weird.* Then it hit me. *Would he do it?*

He talked about it quite a bit after his diagnosis, but he talked about many things that he never did. Still, my mind raced. *If he's going to do it, where would he go? How would he do it? How would I find out? How could I shelter the kids? What would I tell them? Would I stop him if I could? Or would it be for the best? Will the last thing I ever say to him be, "What the fuck are you doing?"*

The kids distracted me, and before I knew it, it was time to head to school and work. I glanced out the window and saw Russ in the detached garage at the back of our lot, still avoiding us but safe. On my way out of the neighborhood, I checked the security cameras on my phone. He was in the house, and he was fine. We all survived to live another day.

2

Seeing the Signs

I tried to think back to when it began. I analyzed everything that seemed out of place, that didn't make sense. But in the stress of life with two young kids, who knew what was normal?

Ryan was born in 2010 and Hailey in 2013, and a whirlwind ensued. Each addition to our family brought new joy but also its share of challenges.

Ryan was the most adorable and smiley baby, but he was also colicky. And not a little colicky, but the crunching, squirming, squealing kind of colicky. He writhed in pain for hours a day, typically after feeding. We tried changing my diet. One by one, I gave up dairy, gluten, leafy greens, and the absolute worst—coffee. We tried mixing breastmilk with different formulas. It got a little better, but the colic never went away fully until he grew out of it.

He was also terrible at breastfeeding. I jokingly called it "falling asleep at the titty bar." After thirty seconds of feeding, he fell fast asleep and left me with one of two choices. Choice #1 was to sit there, immobilized while he slept. Any attempt to move or place him down would wake him in a fit of tears because guess what? He was hungry. Choice #2 was to wake him up. In this scenario, I got the fit of crying immediately, calmed and soothed him, and convinced him to eat. Then, thirty seconds later, he fell asleep and repeated the glorious cycle.

He loved the bottle and downed the largest nipple size I could justifiably give him for his age. Eventually, I gave up on breastfeeding and entered the worst of both worlds, pumping *and* bottle feeding. I remember days on maternity leave when it felt like half my day was either attached to a machine or washing a thousand little plastic bottle parts. The entire top rack of my dishwasher overflowed with little milk contraptions. Wash. Pump. Feed. Repeat.

Fortunately, Hailey was a bit easier. She wasn't colicky at all and breastfed beautifully. Her infant stage was much saner, partly because of her and partly because I was a more seasoned and less anxious mother. The biggest stress she added was sleep deprivation. Since Ryan downed huge bottles before bed, he slept through the night around six months. Hailey's breastfeeding gift came with a downside—she was nearly a year old before sleep became predictable. Fitful sleep ruled the night, and tiny people ruled the day. I was tired.

On top of motherhood, I worked full time in a high-tech medical device startup. I joined the company when I was six months pregnant with Ryan. Why not take on a demanding new job right before a major life change? I asked my new boss for two days off before coming on board.

"I know you want me to start right away," I said, "but I have to find a daycare for when this kid pops out."

Russ agreed to be Mr. Mom and watch Ryan three days a week, but I knew my husband well enough to know that five days home alone with an infant was not his thing.

By the time I was pregnant with Hailey, I'd been promoted to the Vice President of Research and Development. The company transitioned from a manual surgical device company into a robotics company, a massive change for a small company in Research Triangle Park, North Carolina. We didn't have the pool of robotics talent in the area like in Silicon Valley or Boston. But determined to make it happen, we used consultants to bridge the gap. I expanded R&D from a small group of mechanical engineers into a team of over fifty with expertise in software, electrical engineering, and controls. It was a hectic time, and every day brought a new challenge.

The company went public through a reverse merger in August of 2013. Apparently, being six months pregnant was a signal for significant changes in my career. Going public was a bigger change than I anticipated. Conference calls filled my maternity leave as we prepared for board meetings—corporate strategy and breastfeeding, what a great combination. The company continued to grow, and attention and responsibility followed. I learned and grew in ways that only startups can offer.

While I drowned in to-do lists, Russ grappled with the dramatic change in his life—high-paid startup executive to chief baby spit wiper. He did his best to be Mr. Mom, but the stimulation I enjoyed each day at the office was a notable void in his life. He'd once been the guy who fixed the most complex problems, both technical and business. But without daily puzzles to solve, the spark that propelled him seemed to languish.

And like most new parents, adult time didn't exist. Every time we tried to be intimate, a cry rang out on one of the baby monitors. We'd arrange a date night, and one or both of the kids got ear infections. Parenthood changed our lives, and we were no longer at the center. We powered on and hoped that, over time, the strain would ease.

So, with massive life changes all around, I couldn't pinpoint the genesis of our struggle. We started therapy when I was pregnant with Hailey. We sat parallel on a couch ridiculously low for my round midsection, and I used the time as a way to vent my increasing resentment.

"It's so freaking frustrating to come home after working all day to see the dishes from the night before *still* in the sink. You say you'll do them in the morning, and you don't. And it isn't because you're watching Ryan. He's been in full-time daycare for years because you couldn't handle him. I don't know what you do all day, but thirty minutes to do *something* that helps me doesn't seem like a big ask."

He shot back immediately. "You have no idea what I do. I work all day in the yard, and you don't even notice! Everything I do, you take for granted."

"What about all the things I do?" I asked. "It's not like I'm sitting on the couch eating bonbons. I'm busy all day from 5:00 a.m. until at least 11:00 p.m.—every day! And, yes, I know you do a lot of work in the yard. But yesterday, you spent *all day* reloading pistol ammo! Couldn't you have stopped an hour early to clean up? Make dinner? Something that helps the family?"

He rolled his eyes. "Reloading keeps my brain engaged. I like the science and methodology behind it. Without that, I'm nothing but a nanny and landscaper. I didn't work my ass off all my life to sit around and do nothing."

"It's not nothing. It's raising a family. You could be spending time with Ryan, teaching him, playing with him. We can't get this time back." I paused to collect my thoughts. "Besides, you barely even shoot anymore. You used to go to matches with your friends all the time, but now, you always make an excuse not to go."

"Well, I won't go to Darren's because the last time I saw him, he barked orders at me like a dog. And Mike, he took my money for shells and never gave them to me. They're all a bunch of assholes."

I'd heard this so many times that it felt like a record on repeat. "You know, with you, everyone is an asshole. When *everyone* is an asshole, you may want to take a step back and consider that *you* might be the asshole."

We went to therapy for almost a year. It helped a little. The dedicated time to talk about us was a start. Our therapist gave us tools to see each other's side, to communicate better. But we got stuck in the same circular patterns—argument after argument.

One of the things I used to adore about our relationship was that we never argued. We were engineers and preferred to work with data and facts. Both of us managed large teams at work and knew how to handle difficult situations. When we disagreed, we talked it out logically. Sometimes, one of us thought it out better than the other. The compelling case won, and that was that. More often, we both made good points, and we merged our ideas. Our joint solution surpassed the sum of the parts. It was easy and empowering.

Time after time, we'd faced adversity as partners. We moved cross country twice together—no fighting. We designed and built a house in the middle of the housing market collapse of 2009. Our builder went out of business before he finished and left us with liens on our property and a long punch list to complete on our own—still no fighting. We navigated career changes, me going back to school full time, building a life in North Carolina, and instead of fighting, we worked as partners.

But not anymore. Everything seemed like a struggle. One time while we spiraled down another fruitless argument, I had an epiphany. Our logical dialog was gone. Russ didn't listen like he used to. I stopped and blurted, "It's like you're arguing just for the sake of arguing. What you're saying doesn't even make sense."

He stormed off and spent the night in the guest room.

By 2015, the arguing was unbearable. In his depression and anger, Russ turned to alcohol for relief. He picked up the kids from daycare in the afternoon, and by the time I got home at 6:00, he was on his second or third drink. After dinner, he passed out on the living room couch. If the kids made any noise, he barked and stormed off, either to the garage or to the guest bedroom. We tiptoed around to avoid disturbing Dad. Even our living room didn't feel safe.

I realized I couldn't live my life—or raise my kids—in that environment. I searched Zillow for rentals. While he dozed in his drunken stupor, I envisioned escaping to a place where we didn't walk on eggshells. A place to giggle and laugh without repetitive battles to nowhere.

In September of 2015, I scheduled an appointment to view a townhouse nearby. It had everything we needed: separate bedrooms, a nice kitchen, a play space. It even had a fenced yard in case Russ let me keep one or both of the dogs. I left work early to meet the realtor, but doubt surrounded me. *Can I do this? I've been with him for so long. Can I leave him? Can I raise the kids on my own? Has it come to this?*

I waited for over an hour, but the realtor didn't show. I was about to leave when she finally called back. She apologized, but my raw nerves and aggravation were apparent. I'd canceled a meeting at work to be there, and for what? I still hadn't seen the house, and now, I'd be late getting home. I wondered what hell that would unleash. She sensed my distress and gave me the lockbox combination.

When I opened the door, I entered an alternate universe. Unlike our beautiful house with natural light and handpicked modern decor, the townhouse was dark, dingy, and smelled like something unidentifiable. Folds in the carpet promised weekly face plants, and each turn uncovered a new mess—or worse, a new smell. *This isn't the life I envisioned. This isn't the life I want.*

On the drive home, I prepared for the worst. *Keep the kids calm. Make dinner. Watch TV in the bedroom. Get them to bed. Finish your slides for the Board. Go to sleep.*

But, to my surprise, I found joy in the house. Russ and the kids were watching Bugs Bunny. They laughed and joked when Yosemite Sam fell for another silly trick. Russ had made dinner and put it in the oven to keep it warm. I hugged everyone and took in the scene. It was perfect. I felt foolish for how I'd spent the last two hours. *Maybe I was overreacting? Maybe we could be happy?* I was as confused as a battered wife grasping her apology flowers.

Every introspective moment, I tried to visualize the rest of my life. Would I leave Russ and raise the kids alone? Would our divorce be horrible like his first one, or would we settle things amicably? Or maybe we'd figure out how to make it together. Maybe we'd come back together as our kids became less demanding, less needy. I couldn't predict the outcome, but I knew something had to change. The data was clear. But like in engineering, as soon as I thought I'd figured it all out, new pieces of data emerged that changed everything.

It was early 2016, and the company I worked for had acquired a new robotic system that immersed me in harmonization plans. Doctors used the device clinically in Europe, and we wanted FDA approval for use in the United States. It was an enormous project, and the executive team decided that I would lead it. Gantt charts and design documents covered my desk when my cell phone rang. It was the monitoring company for our security system at home. Something triggered the alarm, and they wanted to know if it was a mistake or the real deal.

"I have no idea. I'm not home," I snapped, a little annoyed and a bit concerned. I looked at my watch. "This is the time my husband usually gets home with the kids, so it's likely okay. Assume all is fine, and I'll call you back if it's not."

Before I hung up, another call came in. It was Russ. When I answered, I could hear the alarm blaring.

"What's going on?" I asked, trying to discern his voice from the chaos in the background.

"This fucking alarm system won't work!" he screamed.

I sighed as I pictured two wide-eyed kids staring at him. I couldn't get him to stop swearing. My Boston heritage blessed me with a horrid potty mouth, but I never cussed with the kids around. I'd pleaded for him to stop, but the profanity still flowed.

He went on, "I'm punching in the code, and nothing is happening. This thing is a piece of shit!"

I took a deep breath. "Enter the code in slowly. Sometimes, you go too fast." He was a guitar player with fast fingers, and the alarm often failed to comply with his speed.

"I've tried. It's not working. We need to call the company and get them out here to replace this thing."

I heard the rage rising in his voice and thought of the kids. Screaming alarm. Screaming dad. Tears building. My evening would be a blast.

"Try it one more time. 6 - 8 - 9 - 4 - 2 - OFF. Do it at that pace."

"I'm telling you this thing doesn't work. I've tried it a dozen . . ."

Suddenly, the alarm shut off, and calm ensued—like the eye of a hurricane.

"Okay," I said. "That was fun. Are the kids all right?"

"Yeah, they're fine. But we have to get this piece of shit replaced. It's unacceptable."

Usually, Russ handled broken things at the house, but somehow, it became my responsibility. His list never got done, so I piled it on top of mine.

"I'll take a look when I get home. Do you want me to leave now?" I asked.

"No, I'm fine. That thing is so loud. It hurts my ears and makes my head feel like it's going to explode. I'll see you later."

When I got home, I checked the alarm as soon as I walked in. Everything seemed fine. The code worked; the buttons registered. It was like it always was. Something seemed off with the entire situation, but I couldn't quite figure out what. *Did he enter the code too fast? Something feels odd.*

Two days later, it happened again. Then again the next week. Now, I was paying attention. I needed more data. More facts. *Keep your eyes open, Nicole.*

Then we were watching the news before the standard rush-to-school routine. While pouring my second cup of coffee, I threw my typical breakfast, Ezekiel bread, in the toaster oven. A few minutes later, a loud popping noise came from the kitchen.

"What the hell was that?" Russ asked as he jumped to his feet.

"It's just the toaster. The pan on top warps when it heats up. I should throw it away, but I still use it for Hailey's chicken."

He sat down, but a confused and concerned look lingered. As I sipped my coffee, uneasiness flooded my mind. *Odd. That damn pan pops every morning. I mean every—single—morning. It's as common as the coffee we drink. Hasn't he noticed? But he notices everything. Doesn't he remember?*

The question hit me hard. Didn't he remember the pan popping every morning? Didn't he remember the alarm code? Seven years of the same code, and we'd never had a problem. I still couldn't reproduce his issue. Was he punching in the wrong code? It didn't seem possible, but I didn't have another logical explanation. *Keep watching. Keep observing.*

Another day, I heard him grumble after I put the kids down to bed.

"What's wrong?" I asked.

"It's this damn TV—and Ryan. Ryan always leaves the TV on this stupid DVD, and I can't figure out how to get it back to the news. He needs to stop touching this shit."

I tried to calm him down. "You have to hit the source button and then toggle over to HDMI1. From there, you can change it to the channel you want."

Again, odd. Russ was a computer scientist and electrical engineer. He'd set up the routers and all the devices in our house. He had twenty-four plaques hanging in his home office, each displaying one of his patented inventions in either microprocessor or internet technology design. Yet, he couldn't change the source on the TV, a task that my five-year-old son could do. Why didn't I notice this before? Something was seriously wrong.

Within a month of that first blaring alarm call at work, I knew my problem was more than Russ being an asshole. He forgot things. He misplaced things. The depression and drinking weren't the cause; they were symptoms. He was sick. He was very, very sick.

Convincing Russ

April 2016

For days, I tortured myself. I knew it would lead to an argument. Russ was a walking hair-trigger, so telling him he was losing his mind certainly wouldn't go over well. I wasn't sure how to approach it. How could I start the conversation? "Honey, I know you think you're right, but you're actually wrong. You can't think clearly because you're sick, and it affects your brain." It made sense to my engineering mind, but it probably wasn't the best approach.

I needed to time it well and broach the subject when he was calm, more like himself. But finding that window with a two and five-year-old around wasn't a simple task. I tried to plan it. I tried to script it out. In the end, like much of my life, it just happened.

It was the spring of 2016. Ryan was in kindergarten but was on a three-week break, or "track-out," that came with his year-round school calendar. I'd researched all sorts of track-out camps, but he ended up back in his old daycare. Hailey was still there as well, and a single pick up and drop off beat driving all over creation. Russ was on afternoon taxi duty, and when I got home from work, he met me in the garage before I even parked the car.

"You wouldn't believe the shit that happened today," he snapped.

I braced myself. I had no idea what to expect at the end of a sentence like that.

"When I picked up Ryan from daycare, the teacher—you know, the one with the thick accent—she read me the riot act about Ryan's behavior. She called him disruptive and said he wouldn't stop fooling around with other kids. She tried to get him to calm down, but he got angry and kicked a chair over. He kicked a chair over! Can you believe it?"

I tried to stay calm to balance his agitation. "Did you talk to Susan, the other teacher? Danika isn't a fan of Ryan, and she tends to be hard on him. Usually, Susan is pretty balanced, and I get a better picture from her."

"No, she wasn't there. And that other teacher belittled me in front of all these other parents and told me how messed up my kid was. It was embarrassing! And Ryan, he's exactly like my older brother, Ray. If we don't do something, he'll turn out to be a complete sociopath."

Ugh. I hated it when Russ compared Ryan to Ray. He was nothing like Ray.

"I think that's a little dramatic," I said. "What are the kids doing? Are they watching TV?"

"Yes, of course. That's all they do," he retorted.

Well, if you put the TV on, of course, they will watch it. I pulled out of the argument rabbit hole and came back to the issue at hand. Then, it came to me.

"There are cameras at the school. We can go back and watch the recording and see what happened." I paused and reached for his hand. "Let's relax and have dinner. We'll talk to Ryan, and I'll talk to Susan in the morning. I know he struggles to behave, but something doesn't feel right. I've never seen him kick anything over."

"Whatever," he said and jerked his hand away. "I'm telling you that kid is a problem. And I can't sit there and have dinner with *them*."

He said the word "them" with such disgust it felt like a baseball bat to the face. They were not "them." They were *us*. These were *our* kids. He went on.

"I'm going for a bike ride. You do whatever you want. You always do."

Another bat smack. I was barely two steps from the car, my briefcase weighing on my shoulder. *Welcome home, honey.*

At dinner, I began the investigation. "Ryan, what happened at school today? Dad said you got in trouble and were upset?"

Ryan looked at his plate and shoved his food around.

"Ryan? What happened?" I repeated.

He looked up and then blurted, "I was playing with my friends during story time, and Ms. Danika told me to be quiet. Then I talked again, and she made me sit by myself *forever*. I missed out on all the activities, and I would have missed outside time if Ms. Susan didn't come back."

I took a breath to figure out how to respond. Daycare and then kindergarten had become a struggle. I hated the constant corrections, but I couldn't let his behavior go unaddressed.

"Well, you aren't supposed to talk when the teachers talk. And she also said you kicked a chair? What happened there?"

"It wasn't fair!" he shouted. "I sat in the chair all through activity time, and when it was time to go out, Ms. Danika said I still had to sit. I got angry, so I kicked the chair."

"Did you kick it over?" I asked.

"No! I only kicked the leg. The chair was fine."

"And what happened then?"

"Ms. Susan came back. She talked to me for a while and then let me go outside."

I stared at his chubby face and bought time to respond. "Well, you know I can watch the video and see exactly what happened. Is there anything else you want to tell me before I do that?"

"No," he said.

I saw the frustration on his face. Red lights, frowny faces, demerits, extra parent-teacher conferences—we'd seen them all. Energy radiated from his antsy little body, and teachers often struggled to keep him on task. My brother was the same way and ended up with an ADD diagnosis later in life. I wondered if the same issue affected our son.

I smiled and tried to put him at ease. "All right. Let's see if we can have a better day tomorrow. Please, don't make the teachers repeat themselves, okay?"

"Okay," he said.

After the kids went to bed, I logged into the daycare portal. I sorted through hours of feed to find the offending incident. Ryan's account was pretty accurate. He sat in the chair for twenty-four minutes—an eternity for a five-year-old boy. Then Ms. Danika came over, and he stood up. After about thirty seconds of back and forth, he flailed his arms and kicked the leg of the chair. Yes, it was a kick, but not even close to kicking over the chair. It wasn't appropriate, but was it appropriate to make a five-year-old sit out for twenty-four minutes? What kind of redirection was that? I made a plan to talk to Danika in the morning and maybe even the director. My kid wasn't an angel, but there were better ways to handle him.

Russ went straight to the basement to reload ammunition after his bike ride. Now that the kids were in bed, he emerged. Despite all the time avoiding us, he still seethed.

"So, what did you find out?" he said, half asking, half barking.

"Well, look at this," I pulled up the video. "Ryan talked during story time, and Ms. Danika made him sit in the chair for twenty-four minutes. When he got up for recess, she told him to sit back down, and he got upset. Here, this is him kicking *over* the chair."

Russ watched the video over my shoulder. "What? Is she serious?" In an instant, all of his anger toward Ryan turned toward his teacher. "That's barely a kick at all! You should have seen the way she treated me. It was demoralizing—and for that? That's ridiculous!"

"I know. I'm going to talk to Ms. Danika and the director in the morning and figure out better ways to manage Ryan. Susan does so well with him. She gives him jobs and things to do, so he feels helpful. Half the time, I think he's bored."

Russ went on like he didn't even hear me. "I'm going to talk to the owner and get that woman fired. She has no business around kids if she treats them that way."

Given his mood, I wasn't surprised he went straight to the nuclear option. I opted for more diplomacy.

"I agree Danika didn't handle it well, but I think we can take care of it more directly. He does cause problems in class, and we have to figure out how to manage it better."

"No, I'm sorry, but that woman is a problem. You should have seen the way she belittled me. She has a chip on her shoulder and needs to be out of there."

As he continued to yell, I felt the stress rise. It was almost 9:00, and I was tired from work, tired from him, tired from everything.

"Well, let's sleep on it. I can talk to the owners in the morning when I drop them off." I had no intention of talking to the owners, but I didn't want to fight anymore.

He sensed my deception, and his roaming anger laser-sighted on me. "Yeah, sure you will. You always say you will. I'm too stupid to handle it, so you will, but then you don't."

"I never said you were stupid. I only said I'd take care of it when I drop the kids off."

"Oh, you definitely think I'm stupid. I can't do anything right. It always has to be you because everything I do gets fucked up. I'm too hard on Ryan. I can't put away the dishes right. I can't fix the cabinets right. Everything I do, you criticize. Everything I do is wrong."

I lost my composure. "I don't even know how we got here. We were talking about Ryan, and now, we're talking about cabinets and dishes. I don't think you're stupid. I'm trying to help!" I shouted as if it would help him hear, but it only triggered more venom.

"I work my ass off all day, and I get nothing from you! Not a thank you, not a good job, not a 'Hey, it looks nice,' nothing! And when you do notice, it's always what's wrong. This is fucked up. That is fucked up. Everything is fucked up! Nothing is ever good enough for you!" he screamed.

He went on and on, how fucked up I was, how he was never good enough, how it was always his fault. There was truth in some of it, but there was so much more. Finally, I couldn't hold back the swelling tide.

"Stop it! Stop it! I can't take it anymore! Just stop it!" I stormed out and retreated to our bedroom. Unable to think or argue, I sat down on my closet floor and cried.

After a few minutes, Russ came in with concern in his eyes. "Are you okay?"

Of course, I'm not okay. You've been screaming at me since the moment I got home. I've been at work all day, then taking care of the kids, and finally, it's time to relax, and you're screaming. I am definitely not okay! The words raced through my head, but only sobs came out.

"I'm sorry. I didn't mean to make you upset."

I'd seen it before. My complete and utter breakdown triggered a brand-new mood. Like some connection in his brain was lost, and my tears dashed in and illuminated the way. He became the sweet and caring man I married. He sat next to me on the floor and held me. My tears soaked his shoulder, and my body collapsed into his. We sat there for what felt like an hour. I cried until there was nothing left. No more tears to fall.

Finally, I stood up and said, "I'm thirsty. And I need a Kleenex."

He followed me into the kitchen and watched as I made tea. Afterward, we sat on the couch. I looked at him and realized that this was the time.

"Russ, I want to talk about something, and I don't want to argue. I want you to listen. Can you do that?"

His body pulled back, but he was still calm. "I guess."

"I think there's something else happening here. I've been watching and noticing things. I don't think this is us fighting or the kids adding craziness. I think something may be seriously wrong. I think you might be sick."

A look of confusion filled his face. His posture got defensive. I headed off his emotions before they could fester. "Please don't talk yet. You promised you'd listen." He relaxed a little, but not completely.

"There's been so much that doesn't make sense. Confusion over the time to pick up the kids, the alarm going off over and over again, you constantly losing your keys—"

"That alarm is screwed up," he interrupted.

"Please, let me finish. This isn't you, and this isn't us. As someone who loves you more than anyone else in this world, I'm telling you something is *wrong*. You forget things that you never used to, and you're not yourself. I was reading about brain fog and how different infections can trigger it. It can be disorienting and gets much worse if you don't treat it. I think it's worth seeing a doctor."

"Why is it always me? Why am I always the one who's screwed up?" he argued, but it was less angry and more heartfelt than before.

I tapped into our year of therapy. "I hear you that I always criticize. I really hear you. I'm sorry that it comes across that way, but I'm constantly busy and tired, and you know that I speak what's on my mind without a good filter." He chuckled as a sign of agreement.

"But I'm not trying to tell you that you messed up the dishes. I'm trying to tell you that I'm concerned because you put the bowl in the wrong place. The same place it's always been and the same place you used to know. I'm concerned because the alarm code still works fine for me, and I can't understand what's causing the problem for you. We need to consider that something is wrong. I think if you search deep down, you'll know that I'm right."

He paused. I could tell he didn't want to believe me, but something in my words hit home. As I saw the doubt in his eyes, I started to cry again.

"I love you," I said. "From the moment I first realized I loved you, I've never wanted to be with anyone but you. This isn't about blame. This is me saying I think you need to see a doctor. You have to admit that things aren't right. Why not cover our bases?" He chuckled again, but tears welled in his eyes.

"Okay. We'll go," he said.

I sat down next to him and hugged him. I was spent, but I felt like I'd accomplished something, like I jumped a big hurdle. And yet, the marathon was only beginning.

4

Finding a Doctor

May-November 2016

I convinced Russ to see a doctor, but the question was, which doctor? I didn't want the typical primary care physician who examined him for fifteen minutes, took his blood pressure, checked his heart rate, ran his cholesterol, and sent him on his merry way. I wanted someone to dig deeper. Outwardly, he was healthy, strong, and fit for a sixty-year-old. That was one reason he never felt old to me even though he was twenty years my senior. When we went for a bike ride or a hike—or even a walk through the airport—I struggled to keep up, not him. We needed a doctor to see past the physical signs and figure out the root cause or causes of his cognitive issues.

In my casual readings on health, I'd come to believe that food was medicine. If we could heal something naturally, without the need for pharmaceuticals, then why not do it? Modern medicine had its place, but it could also be a crutch. Millions of people with Type 2 diabetes took pills or injected insulin, even though diet changes and periodic fasting were more effective. Doctors prescribed three or more blood pressure medications when exercise and weight loss could do the trick.

But Russ exercised and ate well. There was something more sinister behind his decline. A pure naturopath probably didn't have the full toolkit we needed.

Integrative and functional practitioners combined natural methods with more traditional medicine. These doctors typically weren't covered by insurance, but I liked their approach. They spent more time with the patient, ran more diagnostics, took a detailed patient history, treated with nutrition, lifestyle, and supplements when they could, and integrated pharmaceuticals when needed. A colleague at work recommended a practice in nearby Chapel Hill, North Carolina. I'd gone for a wellness check a few months before and was impressed by the experience. It seemed like the best option for Russ.

The first available appointment was two months away, so I used that time to research and assemble a list of questions. At the top of the list was Lyme disease. Russ was a hunter and was always in the woods. He also did all the yard work at the house, and over the years, I pulled at least a dozen ticks off of him. He'd never had a bullseye rash, but I read how Lyme caused brain fog and memory issues, and it seemed like a good fit for his symptoms.

Another top item was heavy metals. Our favorite hobby was sporting clays, which was like playing golf with a shotgun. Russ introduced me to the sport and was an avid shooter and ammunition reloader since his mid-twenties. Each shotshell contained hundreds of little lead pellets designed to destroy clay targets thrown through the air. Lead and other heavy metals kept popping up in my research, and I wondered if Russ's constant exposure factored into his case. I summarized everything on his intake questionnaire and waited for the appointment.

Calling the appointment awkward would be a massive understatement. Russ went back and forth in his support during the days leading up to the appointment. Some days, he was agreeable, and other days, I was being crazy because there was nothing wrong with him. Even as we sat in the waiting room, he asked why we were there in the first place.

Talking to the doctor about Russ's cognitive issues was painful. I saw his frustration rise as I listed the problems. Every example I brought up faced a retort of how it wasn't his fault—or even better, how it was actually *my* fault. At one point, he got so irate that he stormed out to the bathroom. I took the two-minute reprieve as a chance to plead with the doctor.

"I'm telling you, I've known this man for sixteen years, and there's something wrong."

She ran a series of tests to see what she could find. A month later, we returned to review the results. The meeting was unremarkable. Russ's complete blood count (CBC) and comprehensive metabolic panel (CMP) were normal. His lipids and cholesterol were a little low. He should try putting coconut oil in his coffee to elevate his levels. His vitamin D level was low, so she recommended supplementation. B vitamins and folate were normal. His homocysteine was elevated. Did he drink a lot of coffee? Alcohol? Yes, well, he had cut back on that. He was negative for Lyme. The levels of lead and antimony in his urine were slightly elevated, but it wasn't much outside the normal range. All in all, she saw nothing that would cause the cognitive symptoms I described. If we still felt something was wrong, she suggested that we see a neurologist.

When we left the appointment, Russ felt vindicated. He now had ten pages of lab results showing he was fine.

I, on the other hand, felt defeated.

Maybe I am making too much of this? I read that stress caused confusion and memory issues. Perhaps that was the cause? The kids always brought stress, and Russ missed the challenge of a full-time job. His confidence diminished; he was depressed; he was drinking. It all affected memory. Honestly, I forgot where my keys were that morning, and I didn't think that something was terribly wrong. Maybe I was too hard on him. Was I?

It took about a week to regain my resolve. I kept watching. He forgot the time to pick up the kids even though it was the same every day. He misplaced his wallet four times. He couldn't start the weed whacker—twice. He wasn't the man I married. I had to keep digging.

I researched neurologists, but endless Google searches felt more like a maze than an answer. What kind of specialist did we need? Someone who specialized in brain fog? Was that even a thing? Or should I look for a psychiatrist who could address his depression, anger, and drinking?

Then I came across a neurologist in Raleigh who marketed himself as a diagnostician. He covered cognitive and behavioral health and performed an extensive intake appointment. Patients spent a full day at the facility and completed a series of cognitive tests. At the end of the assessment, the doctor gave a diagnosis and referral if needed. Our first foray into medicine only strengthened Russ's resolve. I had one more shot—either uncover the problem or forever be labeled the crazy wife. This intense day was exactly what we needed.

I called and booked an appointment for the day before Thanksgiving. The kids and I planned to go to my brother's in Virginia that day, but if I didn't take the appointment, the next available slot wasn't until January. There was no school, and daycare was only open a half-day, so I asked Ryan's former teacher, Susan, to pick them up and watch them for the afternoon. She'd quit teaching to go back into software development, but her job was flexible, and she missed being with kids. She had bonded to ours and became like an adopted aunt. Since we didn't have any family nearby, her help was a relief valve that we desperately needed.

As we sat in the waiting room, Russ was stiff. He refused to look me in the eye and paced from side to side in the small room. I asked if he wanted a granola bar, an apple, coffee—anything to break the tension and have him acknowledge my presence. All I got was a series of head shakes.

When the nurse came to collect us, she took his height, weight, pulse, and blood pressure. He joked with her but refused to look at me. It would be a long day, so she pointed us toward the bathroom and the water cooler before depositing us in a small room with no windows. Three chairs and a desktop computer on a small table awaited us. Russ finally looked at me, but fear and disgust clouded his gaze. I looked at my shoes, and we waited for the doctor for what felt like an eternity.

When the doctor arrived, he described the details of the day. Most of the work would be on the computer. Russ would perform a series of exercises and tasks to assess his cognitive status. They also had a series of imaging and electrode-based tests that could be useful depending on the cognitive assessment results. I had prepared Russ for this based upon my discussion with the scheduling nurse, so he sat quietly.

As we reviewed his patient history, the nurse instructed me to let Russ answer. Spite covered every word. "Well, *she* thinks there's something wrong with me." Then, "I don't know, why don't you ask *her. She's* the reason we're here." I feigned ignorance to the onslaught. *Breathe in, breathe out.*

When it came time for the first assessment, Russ sat in front of the computer, and I sat behind him in the corner. The nurse told him to follow the instructions on the screen and let them know when he finished. The first section was a little ridiculous. It was multiple choice for basic questions: What year was it? What season was it? What month was it? What town were we in? He didn't even have to type; he only had to click the right answer. With each question, he grew more insulted.

"Seriously? This is your big cognitive diagnostic day? This is a huge waste of time."

"It's only the beginning," I said. "Keep going. We're here, and we're paying no matter what, so we might as well make the most of it." I tried to remain supportive, but doubt rushed in. *What if I'd made the wrong choice?*

He completed a series of exercises, and between each one, we waited. They warned of a long day, but the project manager in me couldn't help but criticize the inefficiency. *Of course, it will take all day if you make us wait forty-five minutes between each exercise. PLEASE get in here and keep this moving so he doesn't storm out.*

I was glad the kids and I were leaving for Virginia the next morning without Russ. He never felt comfortable at my family events, and at some point, I stopped begging him to go. *At least I'll have four days away from him. It will take that long for him to cool off after this.*

After the initial set of simple tests, they started a series of exercises with varied instructions. "You will see a symbol. Then you will see another symbol. If the symbol is the same as the one you saw before it, hit the right arrow key. If it is different, hit the left arrow key."

He turned around and looked at me. "I don't get it."

I repeated the instructions verbatim because they seemed self-explanatory. Russ still looked confused.

"Look, there's a tutorial. Hit that button," I said. Step by step, the program walked through the process showing the symbols that would arise and highlighting the correct and incorrect answers. I was pretty sure Ryan, our six-year-old, would understand it.

"I still don't get it. This is stupid," Russ snapped.

I was taken aback. "Well, give it a try. Hit the go button and follow the instructions. If the symbols are the same, hit the right arrow. If they're different, hit the left arrow."

He hit go, and I watched his entries. Sometimes, he seemed to get it, and other times, he seemed to guess. I wasn't sure what to make of it. He finished the exercise, and similar ones followed.

"Hit the arrow key representing the direction of the object . . . Touch the screen where you see the X . . . See a series of words, perform a task, and click on the words you saw before the task . . . Press the space bar when you see the following pattern." Some of the tests he handled with ease, and others he struggled to understand the directions. My brow furrowed more with each new exercise.

Finally, he gave up. "I don't get this at all. It's so stupid. We're wasting our time. *You* are wasting my time."

I shook out of my thoughts and confusion and turned my attention toward the screen. There was an obvious tutorial. At the top of the screen was a series of numbers. Each number was associated with a symbol right below it. Then, at the bottom of the screen, there were the same symbols in a series. Russ was supposed to enter the number that went along with each symbol. The program didn't even take the key of symbols and numbers off the screen—it was still right there. All Russ had to do was look at the symbol, look at the key above, determine the number that went with it, and type it in. Again, I was pretty sure Ryan could do it.

I tried to explain it in my own words and asked Russ to repeat the tutorial. He was still confused. Eventually, I encouraged him to start the test to see what happened.

When the first set of symbols and numbers popped up, he stared. "I don't know what to do."

"Just enter the number that matches the symbol from the key above." I wasn't sure if I was supposed to help him, but he struggled so much I couldn't stay silent.

He turned back toward the computer and typed. 1 . . . 2 . . . 3 . . . 4 . . . 5 . . . 6.

"Babe, you're supposed to match the symbols with the numbers above. Like that heart goes with a 5, so you type a 5." Now, I'd crossed the line, but I couldn't believe he couldn't figure it out. He had a master's degree in computer science. He wrote lines of complex code with loops and recursion. The exercise was a simple code match. What was going on?

1 . . . 2 . . . 3 . . . 4 . . . 5 . . . 6.

A new set of symbols and numbers popped up, and he entered the same numbers again. And again. And again.

I sat there, dumbfounded. *This is way worse than I thought.*

When Russ completed the exercise, he looked back at me. His confusion with the test collided with the confusion on my face, and he became agitated.

"I don't understand why we're doing any of this. Push the right arrow, push the left arrow, push the space bar. It's all a bunch of shit! None of this is helping me!"

I couldn't break out of my stupor, and he reacted to my raw emotion.

"What's wrong with you? I'm getting out of here."

When he stood up, it triggered me back to reality. I started my usual course of damage control.

"You're probably hungry. I packed a sandwich; do you want that? It's been a long morning."

"I don't want a damn sandwich. I want to get out of here." As he tried to leave, a nurse opened the door and startled him.

"How's everything going?" she asked. She had no idea what she'd walked into.

"I think we're done," said Russ.

"We have a few more tests that we want to run if that's okay," she said calmly.

"No, it's not okay. I'm sick of being locked in here with your stupid computer games!" Russ shouted.

The nurse then turned to me to gather more information. I studied my shoelaces as if they held the answers I needed.

"I'm sorry things aren't going well," she said. "Hey, I noticed you have some shooting magazines there. Are you a hunter?" The nurse changed the subject as if completely ignoring his discomfort.

Russ paused. "Uh . . . yeah. I like to shoot birds mostly. Dove hunting is my favorite."

"My husband *loves* to hunt. He keeps trying to get me out there, but I can't see myself killing anything. I like to shoot, though." She rolled on with the conversation as if they had just met at Starbucks.

"Have you ever tried sporting clays?" Russ asked. "It was invented to mimic bird hunting. Targets fly from all different directions. Incomers, crossers, they even have targets that roll on the ground like a rabbit."

"Oh, that sounds like fun! Where do you go?" she asked.

The conversation continued. Russ talked about our favorite shooting ranges, the types of guns we owned, and typical course rules. I was amazed. The nurse steered him away from his near implosion, right in front of my eyes. He was now calm and confident. He even looked over at me and lovingly described what a good shot I was.

At a natural pause, she asked, "I've got a couple more things that we need to do. Are you game for another exercise?"

"Sure," he said.

Wow. That was freaking amazing. Whatever the hell she did, I need to try it.

The rest of the afternoon passed much like the morning. Some exercises Russ did well, and some exercises he didn't understand. As time went on, he got increasingly irritable. They took him to another room for a series of tests, but he returned frazzled and spent. The nurse's expression let me know they couldn't complete what they'd planned.

It was almost 6:00 p.m., and even I was tired. I texted Susan and asked if she could take the kids to dinner. I hated to impose further, but we couldn't leave before the wrap-up with the doctor. The day's events needed an explanation.

When the doctor finally came in, he had two other people with him, a doctor in training at the clinic and a student. *Great. Just what we need—an audience.*

"Well, Mr. Bell," he said, "We weren't able to complete the assessment, but from what we could do, I can see there's a fairly significant problem with your cognitive abilities. I'd like to order an MRI to see what's going on."

Patience wasn't typically my virtue, and after all day with Russ barking at me, I wanted the doctor to get to the point.

"What do you think is going on?" I asked.

The doctor flipped through a series of fresh printouts. "I can't give you anything definitive without some imaging work, but I'd say there are two contenders. The first is a vascular issue, like a previous stroke or a blockage causing inadequate blood flow to part of the brain. The second is a neurodegenerative disease, such as Alzheimer's." The last word hung in the air like a polluted cloud.

"Alzheimer's?" I questioned. "That doesn't make sense. He has no family history and is so young. He does have high blood pressure and has for years, so the vascular problem is more likely, right?"

The words poured out, but I struggled to think. We'd run out of food hours ago, and I was hungry, exhausted, and dying to get out of the coffin they called an exam room.

"It could be, but I won't know until we get an MRI. We'll get one ordered and can schedule a follow-up. They'll get you all set up when you check out."

And that was it. It was over. After a long day filled with empty pauses, they shuffled us out because it was closing time. I glanced over at Russ, and he looked as stunned as I was. *What just happened? Did he diagnose Russ with a major brain issue and then push us out the door?*

The ride home was silent. I was at a loss for words and was too tired to pretend otherwise. Russ stared out the window, his eyes squinting like he was thinking, but his stare was vacant, like he was in a trance.

Susan and the kids were waiting for us when we got home. It was close to bedtime, so the flurry of activity distracted me from the events of the day. With both kids tucked in, I went downstairs and saw Russ on the couch. The TV wasn't on. He wasn't flipping through a magazine. He was just sitting.

I sat down next to him and held his hand.

"Do you want me to cancel the trip to my brother's? We don't have to go."

"No. Go. There's nothing you can do. We'll wait to see what the MRI says and go from there."

We sat in silence for a bit, and then I said, "You know, I love you. I love you no matter what. We'll figure this out and get through it, okay?"

I tried to project strength even though I felt my mind crumble. I wanted answers, but I wanted those answers to be more straightforward. Easier.

"I love you too."

Then he paused and looked at me; the outer corners of his eyes turned downward. I recognized the expression. It was how he looked when he shared his most introspective thoughts. It was a face that was hard-won, then commonplace, and now elusive.

"Thank you for all you've done to help me," he said. "I know I'm an asshole most of the time, and you don't deserve that. I'm so sorry." Tears formed on his face. "I guess I was just scared—scared that you might be right."

I held on to him, and we both cried.

5

The Funeral

December 2016

It was a pretty typical Saturday, and the morning started with a basketball game. I coached Ryan in the five- and six-year-old bracket and spent most of the session screaming, "Dribble! Don't forget to dribble!" or, "No, not that way . . . the other way!" I loved coaching and teaching the kids my favorite sport, but I always left games feeling like I needed a cigarette—even though I didn't smoke.

Russ couldn't handle the noise. Games were played on a half-court, meaning that the small gym housed two cacophonous games in every time slot. Other common shouts of coaching wisdom included, "That's not our whistle . . . keep going!" or, "Don't worry about what they're doing, play *our* game!"

Russ had volunteered to save his eardrums and stay home with Hailey. She found Elmo much more interesting than basketball anyway. When we got home, Russ had a weird look on his face.

"I got a call from Camilla," he said.

I was surprised. He had a contentious relationship with his ex-wife, and she never called him unless it was something urgent about their daughter, who wasn't that much younger than me.

"That's weird. Is everything alright with Alyssa?"

"Yeah, Alyssa is fine. It was about my dad. He died yesterday." His face looked blank. He never got along with his dad, but I could see the shock.

"Oh, babe . . . I'm so sorry. Wait, why did Camilla call you? Why didn't Doug call you?"

Russ hadn't talked to his little brother in a while, but I figured their father's death would be enough to break the ice.

"I don't know. I guess he's still pissed at me, although I'm not sure why. Camilla found out through my cousin and called to give her condolences. She was surprised I didn't know."

"Do you know when the funeral is? Are you going to go?"

The answer to the last question would be a no-brainer for most people, but I wasn't so sure for Russ. He harbored immense anger toward his dad that he couldn't move past. He blamed his dad for not protecting his mother when a neighbor harassed her. He blamed his dad for not protecting him and Doug from the abuse of their older brother. There were long, complicated stories and years of therapy, but no resolution.

"I think I will go," he said. "The funeral is on Tuesday, so I may drive down to Atlanta and spend Monday night with John. It would be good to catch up with him and Eleanor."

John was an old friend of Russ's from when he used to teach electronics. I'd met him and his wife Eleanor when we stayed at their house during our cross-country honeymoon adventure. John was a lifelong friend, and Russ hadn't seen him since that trip over ten years ago. I knew some quality time would be good for him.

"Do you want me and the kids to go with you?" I asked.

The offer was genuine, but its reality made me wince. First, there would be sixteen hours round trip in the car with a three- and six-year-old. While it would be nice for them to meet John and Eleanor, I pictured Hailey wailing over something, Russ getting angry, and me craving a vodka tonic before we even left North Carolina. And then there was work. For some sadistic reason, major deadlines loomed at the end of the year, and the month before the holidays promised pure chaos. Back-to-back meetings and a growing list of action items filled my week. Then, of course, it was almost Christmas. My parents planned to fly into town on Wednesday. I had to go shopping, clean the house, and the tasks multiplied.

"No. The trip would be no fun for the kids, and I don't think I can handle them in the truck anyway. If I go, I'll go alone. It will be quick. In and out."

I wondered if the pained look on Russ's face was because his dad had died or because it was now official—his dad would never meet our kids. We'd talked about a trip to go see him, but the pull wasn't strong enough to make it happen. Our kids and Alyssa were the only grandchildren. A wave of guilt overcame me. *I should have forced the issue. We should have made the trip.*

Then another emotion took over. Fear. Would Russ be okay to drive all that way on his own? A lot had changed in Atlanta since he lived there. Could he navigate on his own? I struggled to speak the question.

"Are you sure you don't want me to go and help drive? Atlanta traffic is brutal, and there's always construction."

"No, it'll be fine," he replied. "Getting to John's is easy, and I'm sure he'll go with me to the funeral. I have the GPS if I need it."

Usually, I wouldn't be the least bit concerned. Russ had a fantastic sense of direction. I'd seen him drive by the seat of his pants in places he hadn't been in years. But we were still awaiting the MRI results. I had no idea what plagued his brain.

He sensed my concern. "Don't worry. I'll be fine." Then he paused and flashed a sly grin. "Plus, don't forget, you're terrible at directions. You'll just get me lost."

I laughed because I knew he was right. In my early twenties, I realized that my sense of direction was atrocious. Unfortunately, that realization came after many misguided escapades where I'd convinced myself and others that I knew the way. Right or wrong, I wasn't confused. After a dozen or so bonus adventures, I finally conceded to my broken internal compass.

"Well," I said, "We have another day or two, so I can always move things around if you change your mind."

On Monday morning, Russ left for Atlanta about the time I left to take the kids to school and daycare. I checked on him throughout the day, and everything seemed fine. Then, during an afternoon meeting, he texted to let me know he'd arrived at John's. I was relieved. *That was the hard part. John will get him to the funeral, and then getting home is easy.* At least Russ's navigational skills were still solid.

Tuesday morning, I called to check in. Russ had been up late drinking with John and Eleanor, so he sounded tired.

"Is John going to the funeral with you?" I asked.

"Yes, but I'm following him there. I want to head home after the service and get a few hours of driving under my belt before it gets too late. I can stop somewhere, find a hotel, and then finish the drive in the morning."

I hesitated. "Are you sure? Don't you want to spend some time with Doug or your friends? There's no rush to get back."

"Screw Doug," he snapped back. "He didn't call me, so he obviously doesn't want to talk."

I cringed. Doug was the only one in his family with whom Russ was close. His mother had passed away years ago, and his older brother—who he hated anyway—had passed two years ago. Doug was a lot like Russ, and they always had fun when we got together. *He keeps pushing everyone away.*

Later that afternoon, Russ texted that he was on his way home and promised to call when he stopped at a hotel. As the kids settled down to watch TV before bed, my cell phone rang.

"How did it go?" I asked.

"It was fine. It was actually a nice service. I'm tired, though. Been a long day."

I heard the fatigue in his voice. No matter what anger he held, saying goodbye to his dad had to be tough.

"So, what happened with Doug? Did you talk to him?" I hoped it went well so the kids would get their uncle back.

He scoffed. "Barely. He asked what I was doing there and then walked away. After that, I sat in the back and left after the service was over."

Yikes. It was worse than I thought. Russ's dad had dementia at the end, and caring for him was rough. Doug managed everything, even though he was also battling throat cancer. It must have been quite a mess for things to get that bitter between him and Russ. Doug didn't know about Russ's problem. Russ made me promise that I wouldn't tell him, or anyone else for that matter.

"How far did you get on the drive?"

"I don't know. I'm not too far out of Georgia. I got hungry, so I stopped early and grabbed something to eat. Now, I'm settled in with the mini-bar."

His comment reminded me of when Russ and I used to work together. Instead of venturing out for dinner, we ordered room service and raided the mini-bar, happy to have sequestered time to explore our budding relationship. The memory made me smile.

"I'm jealous. Work has been insane and then the kids. I could use a nice drink and some quiet right now. But instead, I get to do personnel reviews after I put the kids to bed. My favorite."

He laughed. He once managed a team of about seventy-five people, so he knew the fun ahead of me. I hedged my complaints and thought about the stress of his day.

"Are you doing all right, really?" I asked.

"Yeah, I guess," he said with an unconvincing tone. "Being back home sucks—so many bad memories. And seeing Doug kind of sucked too. I'm not sure what to do about that one. But most of all, I'm tired."

"Then get some sleep, and we'll see you tomorrow."

"Will do. Love you."

"I love you too. Sleep well."

The next morning, a text announced that he was on the road again. I did the quick math and figured he'd be home sometime around noon.

I went about my day without any thoughts of his trip. My parents were arriving later that evening, and I had errands to run after work. Between meetings, I wrote shopping lists and made last-minute Christmas orders. Then, around 4:00 p.m., Russ called. I was waiting for a phone call from a consultant, but I answered to make sure Russ was picking up the kids.

He sounded distraught. "Hey, um, something's not right here. I need you to come get me."

I was confused. "Come get you? Get you where? Aren't you home? Is the truck okay?"

"Yeah, the truck is fine, but something's wrong. I'm at a gas station. Can you come?"

A gas station? A gas station where?

"I probably can, but I need to know where you are. What does the GPS say?"

"I can't tell on this piece of shit. Half of the roads aren't even there."

I wished he learned how to use the GPS on his phone, but he still loved that old Garmin. The maps were out of date, so I didn't doubt their inadequacy.

"I'm at a gas station. There's a Waffle House across the street and a Bojangles right next to me."

I sighed. "Russ, you just described half of the gas stations in the South. Do you see a road sign or an exit number? Are you still on 85?"

"I don't know. I only see the gas station, the Waffle House, and the Bojangles."

I felt as lost as he was. Suddenly, I had a thought. "Why don't you go into the gas station and ask what town you're in?"

"Okay. Hold on." I heard his breath as he walked. Then a slight jingle of the door. "Hey, man, do you know what town this is? What was that? He says it is Braselton."

I pulled up Google Maps and typed in Braselton. "Braselton, Georgia? That's only an hour outside of Atlanta. Are you sure you're in Braselton, Georgia?" *What in the world?*

"Yep, Braselton, Georgia. Can you come get me?"

My mind spun. "Braselton is almost six hours from here. We need to pick up the kids in an hour. I actually thought you were getting them."

I stopped. *Deep breaths. What the heck do I do? Okay, think.* Russ left the hotel right outside of Georgia at 8:00 a.m. and drove ALL DAY. He must have gone north and then, after a stop, taken the wrong on-ramp and headed back south. He drove five or six hours in the wrong direction. This was not good. This was not good at all.

I thought for a minute and then asked, "Do you have a full tank of gas?"

"Yeah, I just got gas. Why?"

I ignored his question and kept talking. "I see where you are on the map, and it looks like you're right next to 85. Do you see any signs for 85 North?"

There was silence for a few seconds and then excitement.

"Yes! Over there. I see a sign for 85 North."

He sounded sure, but I wondered if I could trust any of his responses.

"Okay. I can't come to get you because you're too far away. But all you have to do is stay on 85 North. It will take you through South Carolina and into North Carolina. I can talk you through it and check in on you until you're home, or at least close to home."

"So, I get on 85 North, and then what?"

Anxiety filled a balloon in my chest. He made that trip dozens of times when he lived in Raleigh with his ex-wife. It was so simple even my pin-the-tail-on-the-donkey sense of direction could do it. *Deep breaths.*

"Don't worry about that," I said, trying to sound more confident than I felt. "Get on 85 North, and I'll check in with you all along the way. Plus, by the time you need to get off of 85, you'll be close enough that I can come get you."

As I hung up, I attempted to digest our conversation. *How did Russ drive that far in the wrong direction?* I thought getting there was the hard part, but this was a mess. Perhaps it was the stress? All the drinking? I had no idea. All I knew was that this was not the kind of mistake my husband would make.

I asked my assistant to reschedule my phone call, and in a daze, I sent a text to my mom. I told her Russ was having travel issues, and they needed to take a cab from the airport. Travel issues didn't cover the extent of the mess, but I didn't have the energy to explain when I couldn't even explain it to myself. I left the office to get the kids.

By the time I made the kids a quick dinner, an hour had passed. I told Ryan they could watch TV in my room once they finished eating. They never got to watch TV that early, so he smiled ear to ear, oblivious to the looming problem. To avoid their curious ears, I walked upstairs to my office and called Russ.

"Hey, how's it going? All okay?" I asked.

"I guess," he replied. "I'm driving north like you told me. There's been a lot of traffic, so it's slow going. And this stupid GPS doesn't work, so I have no idea where I am. Are you home?"

"Yeah, the kids are eating, so I thought I'd check in. What do the signs say? What are you passing?"

"I don't know. Let me look. Um, I see Wal-Mart . . . Budget . . . Harris Teeter . . . does any of that help?"

I shook my head. *Does he see those on the side of the road?*

"Not really. What else do you see?"

"Um, a bunch of cars. I can give you license plates. Oh, wait! Atlantic Trucking Company. Does that help?"

License plates? Atlantic Trucking Company? Then it hit me; he was reading the signs on the trucks! *Holy shit, this is bad. Is he having a stroke? Should he even be driving??*

I took a deep breath and cleared my mind the best I could.

"The stuff from cars and trucks doesn't help much. How about the green signs? Do you see any green signs with an exit number or something?"

"Hold on. I see a hospital, and now, I see an exit that says, Lavonia. Should I get off?" he asked.

"No, no, no!" I shouted. "Stay on 85. Give me a minute to see if I can figure out where you are."

I brought up Google Maps on my laptop and searched for Lavonia. It was north of Braselton, right on 85. I breathed a sigh of relief. He was going the right way, and he was about where he should be. Maybe this would work after all. I tried to encourage him.

"You're doing great. Just keep going on 85. Now that I'm home, I can check in with you pretty frequently." Then a thought drenched me with worry. "How's your cell phone? Does it have enough charge?"

"I guess. Let me check." He paused. "It looks like it's getting low. It says 30 percent."

"Do you have your car charger? It's usually in the middle console."

"I don't know!" I must have pushed his frazzled mind too far because he sounded upset. "This thing is a piece of shit. It never works right. I'd have to pull over to figure it out."

"No, don't do that," I said. "Keep going, and we'll deal with it later. But we should get off the phone so we don't drain it more than we need to. Keep driving on the road you're on, and I'll check in every thirty minutes. When it gets close to dark, we can decide what to do about your phone."

I thought of all the things he could do to preserve battery life: turn off the Wi-Fi, turn off Bluetooth, turn off the GPS since he clearly wasn't using it. Then I let out a nervous chuckle. *Or he could just plug it in.* If he can't do that, he can't turn off anything. I had no idea how to interact with this new person on the phone.

Somehow, I drummed up some confidence from deep within and said, "I love you. We'll talk soon."

Over the next hour and a half, I checked in every thirty minutes. The conversation went about the same as it did in Lavonia, but he was still on the right road and drew closer to home. I talked him through his confusion with the traffic and beltline around Greenville, South Carolina. He read me all the signs and kept going. Despite our success, I worried. It was dark, he'd been driving all day, and he was still hours away. I looked for hotels along the side of the road and asked him to stop. I tried to convince him to get a good night's sleep, and we'd resume fresh in the morning. Better yet, my parents would be here, and I could come to get him. But he was emboldened by our progress and wanted to be home. He kept going until suddenly, he couldn't.

He called about 7:30 p.m. He sounded flustered and lost.

"Nikki, I need help. You have to help me. I'm not okay. I'm somewhere off the highway. You *need* to help me."

His repeated pleas sent a chill up my spine.

"All right. Where are you?"

I went to the kitchen computer and pulled up Google Maps.

"Did you just get off the road?"

He confirmed that he did, and I did the math from our last call.

"It looks like you should be near Spartanburg, South Carolina. Have you seen signs for Spartanburg? Do you think that's where you are?"

"Yes, I saw signs for Spartanburg. They were all over the road," he replied. There was no hesitation in his voice, so I hoped his memory was reliable.

"That's good. Tell me what else you see."

"Uh, I see a Waffle House."

Again with the freaking Waffle House. Where don't you see a Waffle House around there? I needed more.

"Good. Good. What else?"

"I see a Burger King. Nikki, I need help. I need you to help me."

I felt my hands shaking as I moved the mouse. "I'm trying to help you. Tell me what else you see."

"I don't know," he replied, "and the battery on my phone, it's red. I'm not sure it will last much longer."

"Have you looked for the charger? It's a black cord that plugs into the cigarette lighter. It should be right in the console." I heard him rummage around and curse. "Did you find it?" I asked.

"No, I can't find it. You need to come to help me. Please . . ."

Then we got disconnected. I called back, but it went straight to voicemail—six times. *Shit. His phone went dead. What the heck do I do now?*

Ryan came out of the bedroom. Their show was over, and it was time to go to bed. I switched my brain out of panic mode and shuttled them through their bedtime routine. I went as fast as I could without letting on that something was wrong. They knew Daddy was supposed to be home. They knew Mommy was on the phone with him a lot while he was on the road. Fortunately, they were still young enough to blindly trust Mommy when I said everything would be all right.

As soon as I closed Ryan's bedroom door, the panic rushed back. *What should I do? What's wrong with him? Is he having a stroke? Where the hell is he?*

Waffle House and Burger King—that was all I had to go on. I sat back down at the computer and searched. There were seven Waffle Houses in Spartanburg County along route 85. Seven. And that assumed he was in Spartanburg and that he'd stayed on 85. Fortunately, Burger King wasn't quite the king it was in my youth. I only saw two Burger Kings near a Waffle House. But they were over three hours away, and I had two sleeping children upstairs. My parents wouldn't land at RDU for another two hours. No one knew Russ was having issues. I had no family nearby. There were people I could call, but how could I explain what the hell was happening? And even if I left now, it would take me hours to get there. He could be anywhere by then. *Breathe.*

I decided to call the Spartanburg police department. I told them my husband was in danger and might be having a stroke. I shared the meager information on his location. They said they would issue a BOLO. *A what?* I Googled it. Be on the lookout. The dispatcher assured me they would send an officer to the suspected locations and let me know if they found anything. I waited. Ten minutes later, an officer called. He canvased the entire area at the first rest stop and saw no sign of Russ's truck. A different officer was heading to the second location. Another fifteen minutes. The first officer called back and said there was nothing there either. The chasm in my stomach deepened.

"Mrs. Bell," said the officer, "The BOLO is active, and we'll call if we find anything. Or, if you want, I can issue a Silver Alert and get all agencies looking, including the State Police."

His comment elicited a new level of anxiety. *A Silver Alert? Is that the next move?* Russ needed help, but we hadn't even told our friends that he was having problems. Now, I was going to tell the State Police? Would he be angry at me? He owned so many guns, and I knew he carried one on him. A Silver Alert would put his favorite hobby at risk. Would he ever forgive me?

As I hung up the phone, the armor that had carried me through the day started to crack. The hole inside swelled and pushed into my throat. I couldn't hold it back, and I laid my head on the kitchen desk and sobbed. I let all the pain and strength melt away, and my body convulsed. My nostrils filled, and it became hard to breathe. I was so helpless, so alone.

I pulled myself together and felt a bit of relief that I'd let it all out. But I still needed a plan. I needed advice—a sounding board. Then, it came to me. *Mike.*

Mike was an ex-Raleigh police officer. He'd shattered his ankle while chasing a perpetrator over a fence, and the surgeries that followed never relieved the chronic pain. Eventually, doctors amputated his leg below the knee to provide peace. We'd met Mike through friends and got to know him during the long hours at pistol competitions that Russ and I shot before we had kids. Mike was off the job but was still a good cop at heart. Also, his wife Julie worked as a supervising dispatcher for 911. If anyone could advise me about what to do, it was Mike.

The only problem was, we hadn't spoken to Mike in ages. Russ had gotten angry at him for some stupid bullet purchase, something I'm sure Mike had no idea about and would have immediately cleared up if he did. I tried to get Russ to reach out, but he pulled away from everyone. And Mike had his own struggles. He had a major operation that removed most of his esophagus and left him on a feeding tube for months. Through all of that, we were nowhere to be seen. We didn't go to the hospital. We didn't stop by and bring a joke gift basket as we did after his amputation. Nothing. I made excuses about being busy or blamed it on Russ and his anger, but the reality was that I'd been a terrible friend. As I pressed his number on my cell, I wasn't sure if he would pick up. It was late, and he owed me nothing.

"Nikki?"

Only a few folks who didn't know me at the age of five were allowed to call me Nikki. Despite our relatively new friendship, Mike was in that group.

"I've missed you, lady. How the heck are you?"

And just like that, it was like none of my neglect ever happened. I wasn't sure if I felt relief or more anguish about being such a shit.

"Are you okay?" The cop in him knew that I didn't call out of the blue to catch up on pleasantries.

I explained the situation as best as I could. It was a lot to take in. The last Mike knew, Russ was the group's genius, always with a quippy comeback or joke to make everyone laugh. Would he believe that Russ couldn't find his way home on a highway that led straight back here? Mike had seen a lot in his career and was typically prepared for anything. He listened without judgment, but my judgment crept into my voice. After gathering the facts, Mike said he would talk with Julie and call back.

Within five minutes, my phone rang.

"Nikki, we talked it over, and we think you should issue that Silver Alert. It will get all agencies looking for him since he may not be in Spartanburg at all. If he's had a stroke, we need to find him as soon as we can. I'm dressed, and I think I can be there in a little under three and a half hours."

"Wait, what? Mike, I called for advice, not for you to get in your truck. I have no idea where he is, and it would be the middle of the night before you even got there."

"You can save your breath arguing with me. I'll look for Russ harder than any of those cops, and he needs help. It's non-negotiable."

We hadn't talked to this man in years, and with one phone call, he was out of his pajamas and ready to jump in his truck. My guilt for abandoning him felt even heavier.

"Thank you, Mike. I can't believe you're doing this, but thank you. I'll call you if I hear anything from the cops."

Shortly after the call with Mike, my parents arrived in a taxi. I watched the concern and pain on my mother's face as I relayed the story. Seeing my situation through her eyes only made it worse, and again the armor started to crumble. I had no idea how life had propelled me into that moment. I had no idea how it had gotten this bad, and I hadn't seen it. I let out more of my anguish and tried to ignore how it amplified the pain in her expression.

The police officer from Spartanburg called around 11:00 p.m. They rechecked the exits in question, and there was still no sign of Russ. The Silver Alert was active, and there wasn't much more I could do. He suggested I get some sleep and promised to call with any updates. I checked in with Mike one more time, and he was still en route. He echoed the advice to rest, as did my parents. Sleep seemed impossible, but I forced myself to lie down anyway. Pure exhaustion won over, and before I knew it, it was 3:00 a.m. The phone woke me. It was Mike.

"Nikki, I found him."

"What? How? Where is he?"

I shook off my grogginess and realized that—despite my desire— what happened last night wasn't a dream.

"Turns out there's another exit right past Spartanburg County that also has a Waffle House and a Burger King. The cops were too damn lazy to call the neighboring force. I told you I'd search harder than they would."

I still couldn't believe he found him. "What's he doing? Is he in his truck?"

"No. I found his truck in a hotel parking lot and convinced the clerk to give me his room number. I spent the last hour with him. Nikki, I have to ask, are you guys having problems? He didn't seem to want to talk to you."

"What?" I blurted. "Yes, we're having problems. Things have been pretty shitty, but that isn't what this is about. Mike, he's sick. I've been trying to figure out what's wrong for months, but we're still waiting for the neurologist's results. Something is seriously wrong. He drove for hours in the wrong direction."

Mike seemed skeptical. "He said you messed him up and had him driving for hours. That *you* gave him the wrong directions. He seemed pretty angry. I don't know how to say this without just saying it. Is this whole thing a weird marital spat? He seemed fine when I talked to him. He made sense."

"*I* gave him the wrong directions! Seriously? Mike, no. I'm telling you; he's sick. You should have heard him on the phone. I asked him where he was, and he started reading signs from trucks. He was lost and begging for help."

"Okay, I believe you." But something in his voice made me unsure if it was true.

"Wait, he didn't think it was odd that you showed up at a random hotel in South Carolina in the middle of the night after not seeing you for years? How did he respond?"

"He was confused, but I told him that you sent me. Then he said a bunch of stuff about how you were messing with him."

I was messing with him! I couldn't imagine a version of reality where that was his conclusion.

Mike went on, "He seemed all right, so I left him in the hotel room and told him to get more sleep. I'm in the parking lot now with eyes on his truck. I don't want him to feel like I'm stalking him, so you may want to get down here before he wakes up."

"Yes, you're right. Let me wake up my dad, and the two of us will be there as fast as we can. We should be able to get there before he leaves."

"I'll stay right here until you arrive. You'll see me in the Best Western parking lot across from his truck."

"Are you sure?" I asked. "Don't you need to sleep?"

"I'm fine. Be careful on the drive, and watch out for deer."

I hung up and quickly washed my face and brushed my teeth. As I waited for my dad to get ready, I made a pot of coffee and poured it into some to-go mugs. The adrenaline flowed, but I knew caffeine would be a must after a few hours in the car. While we drove, I filled my dad in on the pieces of the story I'd kept to myself. There was no need to pretend things were normal now. He'd flown into the biggest shitshow yet.

When we arrived at the exit, I saw the sign for the Best Western. I also saw Mike sitting in his truck. He came out to greet me.

"Russ is in Room 109," he said. "I'll wait to see what happens, but I don't want Russ to know I'm here. I told him I was headed home, and if he sees me, it would be weird. I don't want him to feel uncomfortable."

I was in awe. Mike had been up all night, and he was still more worried about Russ than he was about himself. He must have been a damn good cop.

I gently knocked on the door of Room 109 with no idea what to expect. Russ opened the door and peeked through the security latch. When he saw it was me, he closed the door, and for a second, I wasn't sure it would reopen. Then, I heard the latch unhook, and Russ opened the door and stepped aside so I could come in. I went straight to him and hugged him as tight as I could.

"You scared the shit out of me last night," I said. "I was so worried, and I couldn't reach you." I held on to him for a long moment and then bent backward to see his face. "Are you okay?"

"I don't know. I really don't know."

Fear enveloped his face and posture in a way that felt foreign. Russ always knew what to do. His quick thinking mitigated obstacles that others failed to see. When I was scared or lost, he was the rock that restored my footing. Now, it was clear that I needed to be that for him.

"It's all right. I came to get you. My dad is in the car, so we'll drive together in the truck. It's time to get home."

I thought he might argue. Maybe wonder why my dad was there and why I brought him into this. But Russ was quiet and somber. He put his head down and collected his things.

I nodded to Mike on the way out and sent him a text telling him that all was okay. I wasn't sure how I could ever repay him for what he'd done. He brushed off my thanks and told me to be careful driving home. Still selfless. Still thinking about us.

The ride home was silent. Russ asked me to drive, which was unusual in and of itself. Another sign of how displaced we were from our typical lives. As we entered North Carolina, my phone rang. It was the neurologist who was in training that horrible, never-ending day in the office.

"Mrs. Bell, we received the report from the radiologist on Russ's MRI. Is this a good time?"

"I guess it's as good as any. What did you find out?" I asked.

"Well, there are no signs of any vascular damage and no signs of a stroke or any other blockage. In fact, his MRI is pretty normal."

Usually, normal would be great news—a relief. However, the night I just had was anything but normal. "I don't get it," I said. "What does that mean?"

"Well, I'm afraid this makes it more likely that the problem is something like Alzheimer's."

Again, that word. It didn't make any sense. How could it be that word? I had so many questions, but I could sense Russ's tension as he overheard the conversation from the passenger's seat. I tried to stay calm for his sake.

The doctor went on. "I think our next move is to get a PET scan. MRIs are good for structural images, but PET scans focus on metabolism and cellular activity, which is impaired in Alzheimer's. We'll inject a small amount of radioactive glucose into his bloodstream. The scan then provides images of glucose uptake so that we can assess function. There's some paperwork to file with your insurance company, but we'll get that started and take it from there."

As I hung up the phone, Russ spoke one reluctant word. "So?"

"Well, the good news is that the MRI is normal. The bad news is they want to do a PET scan to get more information."

"More information about what?" he asked.

I tried to soften the blow, but my tired brain failed to find words of comfort. "To see if it could be something like Alzheimer's."

I was beginning to hate that word. Then an odd disappointment set in as I realized I was rooting for the stroke.

6

The Wedding

September 2017

It was one of those days when I couldn't get a glimpse of the man he was. I was sitting in the Charlotte airport, trying to get to Shannon's wedding. Shannon was one of my best friends from college. I wasn't even supposed to be in Charlotte. I was supposed to be in Dallas—three hours ago. Hurricane Irma was about to hit Florida, and travel was a mess. Stress brewed because I only had one full day in California, and I planned to meet my plus-one for the wedding, Kathy, in Dallas.

I hadn't been away since Russ's problems had gotten severe, but Shannon was one of my dearest friends. She finally met the woman she adored, and I knew their wedding was an event I couldn't miss. I asked my mom if she could watch the kids—and Russ—for the weekend. Shannon said I could bring Kathy, our mutual friend, instead of Russ since traveling with him would be more work than fun. Everything was arranged, and I was off.

As I tried to figure out how to kill a three-hour layover on a travel plan that was already three hours behind, I received his text. He'd tried to get gas and swore that the new credit card I gave him didn't work.

The nastiness that man could spew in a text message was staggering. You would think I was a captor inflicting him bodily harm, not his loving wife of over ten years. *I'd stolen his money. I'd left him in the middle of a hurricane with no food and no money. This was bullshit.* It went on.

Of course, the hurricane wouldn't hit North Carolina for four more days, if at all. There was plenty of food in the house, and my mom went to the store to get more. None of that mattered. I'd abandoned him. I was the persecutor. The string of text messages told me so.

Maybe he'd forgotten our zip code. Maybe he'd used the wrong card. I couldn't tell, and he wouldn't call me back. Every text message I sent him elicited another nasty response. I sat in a random Taqueria in the airport, barely holding back tears. The weekend was supposed to be my time to escape. My time to relax. So far, it was turning out to be fucking fabulous.

As I analyzed the anxiety building in every cell of my body, I figured out that my biggest fear was being helpless, seeing the impending doom, and not being able to do a damn thing about it. I was an engineer. I liked to fix stuff. I wanted to understand the ins and outs of how things worked and then make them work better, to make people and teams work better. Sitting on the sidelines and watching a catastrophe brew was my worst possible nightmare, and that's exactly where I was. Maybe it was appropriate to figure this out the day before a massive hurricane hit the US. It seemed a good analogy for what raged inside my husband.

The question faced me: How do I react? I could sit there and bawl my eyes out right in the middle of Terminal B. No one would blame me. Half the people who knew about our problem wondered how I skirted daily breakdowns. But what would that help? What would that do? It wouldn't fix anything.

So, in that moment, I turned to my favorite coping mechanism. I sat there and remembered the man he was. The man I loved and lost. I kept the memory of that man alive. He was still with me but gone at the same time. So rather than mourn, I chose to remember.

* * *

Russ and I met when I was twenty-four years old. My MIT adviser had recruited me to work for his new startup company that sought to revolutionize the electronics industry with a new semiconductor material. Revolutions start small, and at the time, we were in a three-room, temporary office north of Boston while the new CEO looked for a larger, more permanent space. Russ walked in for a meeting to learn more about the company. He had a history of pretty impressive executive roles, and in at least one of those, he'd hit it big. One of our board members had worked with him years ago and arranged the meeting.

At the time, there were six of us in the office, with two or three more working in the lab at MIT. One room of the office was used as a conference space, so the remaining two rooms had desks jammed together like a game of Tetris. Since I'd been the last person to join, I inherited the desk by the door. Maybe that contributed to Russ's first impression of me, which was, "Damn, who's that hot secretary?" I guess he was from a different time and era. When I joined the meeting and said something pretty damn sharp, he realized he might have misjudged my talents.

I honestly don't remember my initial impression of him. He was older, shorter than most guys I dated, and had a mustache about twenty years out of date. We didn't have many visitors at the office, so I was curious, but after years of college and now life in that tiny office, I learned to focus on the task at hand and drown everything else out. But once the meeting started, I remember watching him. His presence seemed different from everyone else's. He was charismatic, funny, and extremely confident. Even though he knew nothing about the technology, he asked good questions—strikingly good questions. But he asked them with a slight southern charm that made him seem non-threatening. It was impressive to watch.

A few weeks later, Russ joined the company as the Vice President of Business Development. With him coming on board and other hires brewing, we outgrew the cramped three-room office and moved to trailers outside our new, under-renovation office space in Salem, New Hampshire. I transitioned from my desk by the door to sharing a room with Russ and the CEO. How a kid barely out of college got to sit with two senior executives is still a mystery to me. Maybe looking like the hot secretary had some perks.

I loved being in that office. I listened to their phone calls with investors and customers. I overheard conversations on corporate strategy, and most importantly, I got to know Russ. In fact, when our new state-of-the-art office was complete, I was a little sad. I now had my own corner office with a coveted window, but I missed my officemate.

As we scaled the company, I was in charge of managing our patent portfolio. We licensed the technology my adviser had developed at MIT, and we needed to build upon it quickly to be relevant in the multi-billion-dollar industry we had targeted. That job assignment was the genesis of my love for startups. No other environment would give that kind of responsibility to a twenty-four-year-old with no patent experience whatsoever. But I was a sponge and was surrounded by brilliant people. We developed an invention process that led our small, thirty-person company to file over a hundred new patent applications. The sponge grew.

It became clear that our business model involved licensing to the giants in the electronics industry. That's where Russ came in. He had experience working for and licensing to the giants. He regularly closed multi-million-dollar deals. He was an expert in non-disclosure agreements, joint development agreements, mergers and acquisitions— all of it. He also met the requirements of the company's strict "no asshole" policy.

The only problem was, he was a circuits guy. He had twenty-four patents of his own for things I couldn't even pronounce, but he knew nothing about the material we sold and how it impacted the manufacturing line. He needed a partner who understood the technology at the materials level. He needed someone who knew the patent portfolio's ins and outs and who could speak with customers at their level. It turned out that someone was me.

We spent hours with attorneys developing a licensing strategy. Then we hit the road. Over the next two years, we traveled to California, Texas, Japan, Germany, and France. We went where the manufacturers were, and once we worked our way in, it took months to negotiate deals. I spent more time with him than anyone else, and I loved every minute of it.

Together, we were formidable. Our attorney called me the "steel trap" because I could remember every conversation and immediately think through details in our contracts—the benefits of a young brain. Of course, Russ had the experience and wisdom of what would and wouldn't work in a negotiation. He could also identify the crux of a disagreement and find a solution where both parties got not what they wanted but what they needed. It was masterful to watch.

Somewhere along the way, I realized my interest in him was more than professional. Week after week, we ate breakfast, lunch, and dinner together. To pass the time, we shared our life stories. Our dinners went longer and later. Gradually, his confidence melted away, and I got to know the real him. I felt the pain and loneliness of his childhood and the hours he toiled to break away from his troubled family. I saw the anguish he suffered when his first marriage failed, and he lost all meaningful connections to his daughter. And I understood the work he put into therapy to rebuild and become more self-aware and in control. His age gave him a maturity that didn't exist in my circle of twenty-year-olds, and I was fascinated.

Out of all of his layers, my favorite attribute was his humor. He knew hundreds of jokes and instantly delivered a punch line that matched the situation to a tee. Quips and comments stunned in their wit but soon led to sore sides and clenched knees. My favorites were the ones that cracked him up as much as me. It was like some part of his brain made a hilarious connection, and it took a second or two for the rest of him to catch up. Once it did, he shook with unexpected joy that added to the hysterics. At social events, a gravitational pull seemed to bring people to him. It was almost a given: to find Russ, follow the laughter.

I found myself thinking about him, even when we weren't together. At the time, I was living with my boyfriend of almost seven years. My focus should have been on advancing that relationship. But instead, I thought about Russ. Since Russ was a pathological flirt endeared with southern charm, it was hard to tell when he started feeling the same about me. A look lingered. A smile softened in a new way. An email came at an odd time of night. Our partnership morphed into something different and better.

One evening in France, he walked me to my hotel room even though it was only ten doors past his. When I said goodnight, his gaze pierced through me. I felt the tension and awkwardly repeated my goodnight. As soon as I closed the door, I wished I'd invited him in. But it was complicated. I had officially moved out of engineering and into business development, so Russ was my boss. Plus, he was twenty years older than me. Why did I fantasize about someone who wasn't my type or even in the same life stage? Still, I couldn't help it.

About a week after we returned from France, we were off to Japan. Japanese business hotels were horribly efficient and austere, but Western-style hotels in Japan were fabulous. Modern, sleek common areas invited me in, immaculate rooms calmed my natural disgust for shared bedding, and the IT infrastructure outperformed our office. Other than sushi, which I couldn't develop a taste for, I loved traveling to Japan.

We were negotiating deals with three different companies, and term sheets and long, crowded train rides filled our days. Life in a venture-financed company was fickle, and the politics between our CEO and our founder, my adviser, were getting heated. The CEO wanted us to work against the founder's wishes and sent us instructions—and some deleterious comments—in an email. The email thread morphed into something more appropriate with an action item for Russ. We were jet-lagged and exhausted. When Russ forwarded the email, he forgot that seven emails back, the thread contained comments that sent our founder into a frenzy.

Five minutes after he hit send, Russ's phone lit up. The CEO. The founder. Russ realized what had happened, but he couldn't take it back. Our founder was in Japan and wanted to meet at the hotel. The angst in Russ's face was palpable.

The next several hours consisted of damage control, but it was clear the glass couldn't be unbroken. At the end of a long day, Russ and I plopped onto leather stools at the elegant, back-lit bar. It was time to drink our worries away. I ordered a martini, and he ordered an eighteen-year-old scotch. By the time we decided to call it a night, we were both stumbling and a bit too comfortable. As we walked into the ultra-modern elevator, I tripped on the threshold and fell right into him. He caught me with both arms, and our faces landed within inches of each other.

He gave me a nervous smile and said, "You better be careful. You never know what trouble you could get yourself into."

Emboldened by too much vodka, I stared him straight in the eyes and dared him, "Why? What are *you* going to do?"

He paused for a moment to confirm it was what I wanted, and then he kissed me. Months of tension poured out, and I couldn't wait for the elevator doors to open. I followed him to his room, not able to stop myself from a growing longing.

The rest of the night was the most intense and erotic experience of my life. Until that point, I thought my sex life was good, but at that moment, I realized there was so much more. Russ was a steadfast student of anything that interested him, and sex definitely interested him. He read book after book on the tantric arts, and his passion and experience showed. We devoured each other for hours, with no desire to stop despite our exhaustion. As morning approached, I lay there in his arms, realizing that my best friend had suddenly become the most fantastic lover I ever knew. I was hooked.

In the months that followed, our eagerness to explore each other deepened. Business trips brought new puzzles and challenges during the day and endless lust and sensuality during the night. We ordered room service for dinner and breakfast to extend our coveted time together. As our interest in each other grew, there was no room for anyone else. We wrapped up our flailing relationships and spent every spare moment together.

But as our relationship bloomed, our company crumbled. That fateful email in Japan unleashed a cascade of dominoes. Animosity had always existed between our founder and the CEO, but it became unbearable. Secret board conversations lurked behind closed office doors. Eventually, our founder emerged victoriously, and the board fired our CEO. It shocked most of the company, but Russ and I had seen the events unfold. Russ felt guilty, but he knew he couldn't take back that one simple click.

The next nine months brought two new CEOs. First, our Chairman of the Board stepped in as interim CEO. He sensed that Russ and I were more than colleagues, and before I knew it, I was reporting directly to the CEO and was in marketing instead of business development. Russ guiltily admitted that our new status as peers bothered him. He didn't question my talent, but he had worked hard to get where he was. I was barely twenty-seven and was still wet behind the ears for the role. I admired Russ's honesty and willingness to talk to me about something so uncomfortable. We worked through it in a way that taught me about being a true partner to someone.

Things seemed to be going well until the board hired a permanent CEO. He was arrogant. Brash. I didn't care for him, and Russ was at the point in his career where he wouldn't work for someone he didn't respect. In every meeting and every interaction, Russ looked like a ticking time bomb. He was passionate and opinionated in everything that he took on, and his tumultuous youth taught him all the wrong ways to deal with his emotions. Earlier in his career, he might have made a scene, but years of therapy taught him to control his dissonance. Still, it was there, and in our moments alone, he shared that our future as colleagues was tenuous.

One day, Russ had a two-hour meeting with the CEO. I took an abnormal amount of bathroom trips to monitor the progress, and I knew it wasn't going well. When Russ walked out, he went back and collected his things. As he walked by my office, he gave a two-finger wave and a smirk, letting me know it was the last time he'd be in the building. And that was it. Our time working together was over.

For the next few months, Russ looked for his next gig. He wasn't likely to get another semiconductor job in Salem, New Hampshire, so a move was imminent. For him, that was no big deal. He was born in Georgia and then moved to North Carolina, then California, then Texas, then New Jersey, and then New Hampshire. Moving was a way of life for him. But I was a Massachusetts girl. Most of the people I grew up with never moved more than twenty miles from home. But my friends from MIT were all over the country, all over the world. My brother moved away and lived in Virginia. But most importantly, when I looked into Russ's eyes, it was clear that I loved him. So, when he asked if I would go with him when he moved, I knew the answer was yes.

I went with him to interviews in Maryland and California. We looked at houses. It felt weird to plan such a significant change in a new relationship, but we were best friends. We eventually decided on California. It was a better job for him, and it would be easy for me to get a job in the heart of Silicon Valley. We didn't want to settle there, but three years or so could be fun. Our chairman helped me get a job at KLA-Tencor, a Fortune 500 company in semiconductor equipment.

We were both doing well in our careers. I was coordinating the launch of KLA's flagship inspection station. Fifty percent of my time was in Korea or Japan, and I found that international business travel without Russ was plain old exhausting. I was approaching thirty, and we wanted to get married and start a family. I couldn't imagine life as a new mom when another continent owned half my time. Plus, I missed startup life. The Fortune 500 thing was great experience and training under my belt, but I missed company strategy, board meetings, the stress of fundraising—all of it, good and bad. I liked my job, but the growth curve was shallow and linear. I felt restless.

One night over dinner and a bottle of wine, I lamented over my career. Russ listened intently, as he often did. After a moment of silence, he looked at me and said, "Why don't you go back to school?"

"What? You're crazy. School?"

"Seriously, think about it," he said. "Your degrees are in material science and engineering, and you focused on semiconductors, but you know materials at the fundamental level. You could apply that to anything. Biomedical applications are booming. More and more, they rely on electronics to solve their problems. Go back, get a master's in bioengineering, and retune your career. You're young. It would be easy for you."

I didn't even know what to think about his suggestion. It was so far out of the realm of possibilities; my instincts said no.

"Come on. I'd feel ridiculous on campus with a bunch of nineteen-year-olds. I've done my stint in college."

"Tons of people go back later in life," he said. "And, I have to say, I've found that time with younger people keeps me sharp." He flashed a smile.

He always had a way of making his point while still making me laugh.

"I don't know," I said, sighing. "I can't imagine going back to school after all this time."

He poured two more glasses of wine. "You keep telling me how you want to do another startup. Well, guess what? There aren't a lot of semiconductor materials startups. Too much infrastructure. Bio is where it's at if you want entrepreneurship and a life outside of constant travel to Asia."

He made a good argument. We talked it out until the conversation moved from point-counterpoint to growing and building on the idea. By the end of that bottle of wine, his suggestion had gone from pure crazy to a solid option. He saw the excitement in my eyes and laughed. He knew me well enough to know the seed was planted. Now, he could sit back and watch it grow.

Over the next year, that solid option turned into a plan. I researched programs around the country. Stanford and Duke had programs where I could get a master's degree in a year. Stanford was the easy choice since it was twenty minutes away; however, our desire to stay in California had waned. Russ was frustrated with his new job. He was the VP of Marketing, a discipline for which his company didn't have much respect. He was the fifth VP in a mere six years and was once again ready to do that two-finger wave. Also, we were now officially engaged and wanted to build a family—something we didn't want to do in our three-bedroom apartment or a million-dollar house with an avocado-colored kitchen.

Of all the places to settle, North Carolina was at the top of the list. Russ had lived there before and loved it. Research Triangle Park was budding with young companies and a healthy university culture. The landscape was beautiful, with easy access to the mountains and the beach. And the cost of living was better than other tech hubs like Boston and the San Francisco Bay Area. Once I was accepted at Duke,

Russ found a job with a startup in Research Triangle Park, and we inked our exit from California.

It didn't take us long to start looking at houses and even lots to build on. Pretty early in our search, we found a four-acre lot near a lake west of Raleigh. It had beautiful hardwoods that filled my need for green after all the brown in Silicon Valley. It was in a nice neighborhood where we could build a custom home without homeowner association nonsense. The central location allowed access to most of the Triangle within twenty minutes. But best of all, the back edge of the property abutted the game lands surrounding the lake. Russ could walk right out of our backyard and hunt or fish. We could hike along the ranger trails. It was perfect.

Russ lived in a temporary apartment outside of Raleigh while I finished up work in California for KLA. Every day, he called as he finished up work. One call was particularly memorable. He was having dinner with friends he'd known from his previous stint in the area. I heard them saying hi to me in the background along with the clang of dishes and dinner preparations.

"How was your day?" I asked. It seemed like a good start.

"Well, I don't know," Russ paused as if trying to remember something. "I quit my job and bought that lot." I heard a bit of quip and a bit of nerves in his voice.

"Wait, what?"

So much to digest in so few words. I knew he was butting heads with his new CEO. I wondered if he needed to start his own company because every boss brought more disagreements and challenges. And bought the lot? He now had no job, and I would be in school full time. What the heck?

"I don't even know where to begin," I said. "You bought the lot even though you quit?"

"Yep. You knew that company wasn't a fit. I gave it a try, but I'm too old to dedicate so much time to things I don't believe in. The technology had so many issues, and the CEO was an ass. I figured it was better to call it early. You know what they say, fail fast, right?" He paused. "But that lot is perfect. We've been thinking about it nonstop. I thought I'd take the plunge, and we'd figure it out."

"But, babe, it's such a big decision."

"It's only a lot. We don't have to build right away. I can get another job, you can finish school, then we'll do it. Worst case, we'll sell the lot and be done with it. Are you mad?"

I searched my emotions. All I felt was excitement.

"No, you know I love that place. It's everything we wanted. I can't believe you did it, but I know it's going to be amazing." A wave of warmth came over me. Our new life was beginning.

When we'd moved west, we had a tight timeline and a huge U-Haul trailer behind us. We plowed through and did the entire cross-country trek in about five days. But for our trip east, we had no jobs, nowhere to be, and we were about to be married. The trip became our honeymoon, and we planned our adventure. We pulled out one of those big, paper folding maps and mapped our course: Southern California, Vegas, the Grand Canyon, Zion, Sedona, and more. Every national park nearby got flagged and made our shortlist. We contacted friends and family who lived near our route to see if we could visit.

But the essential part of the journey and the focus of the trip was sporting clays. I was now addicted to Russ's favorite pastime, which was like playing golf with a shotgun. Each course had one to two dozen stations, and each station had two to four targets that flew through the air at different trajectories. Pull the target, lock eyes on it, shoot. The instant gratification of orange targets exploding into hundreds of pieces was exhilarating.

We researched every course from California to North Carolina. Places that hosted national championships, venues with interesting terrain or features, and locations flat out in the middle of nowhere. For weeks, we swapped websites and magazine articles and collected them on the floor of our shared apartment office. When the stack became unwieldy, I organized it in a three-ring binder. Each state filled a labeled tab, and each course became adorned with notes, a map, nearby hotels, and even Walmarts along the way where we could buy ammo. Give two engineers the chance to plan their dream vacation doing their favorite pastime, and apparently, a three-hundred-page binder pops out.

Of course, the first step in an epic honeymoon was the wedding. I had no desire for a big to-do, and neither did Russ, so we decided on a destination wedding. We chose a beautiful resort in Hot Springs, Virginia, nestled in the Allegheny Mountains. It was an idyllic spot for a wedding with stunning views, a fabulous restaurant, two golf courses, a luxurious spa, and—conveniently—two world-class sporting clays courses. On the morning of May 14, 2006, Russ and I shot over two hundred clay targets. That afternoon, we got married, surrounded by a small group of friends and family. I felt unbelievably blessed.

As soon as we got back to California from the wedding, the movers packed up the apartment, and we were off for the rest of our sporting clays adventure. Every course brought new targets with different presentations, trajectories, and speeds. Standard targets were 110mm in diameter, but there were also midis at 90mm and minis at 60mm. The minis were a hoot, and for some reason, my nemesis. There were flat targets in the air called battues and flat targets rolling on the ground called rabbits. Finally, there was the coveted and rare ZZ bird—a standard size target that rested in a two-blade propeller, making it highly unpredictable and super freaking fun.

I was a pretty good shot but still had my moments of utter frustration. In those moments, Russ slowly crept behind me and offered advice.

"You're two feet behind . . . Try increasing your lead . . . Don't stop your swing . . . Your mount is bad. Hit your cheek every time." And if all else failed, "Okay, step back and take a break."

If no one was around, he pinched my nipples to clear my head and make me smile. He called it "Nipple Zen," an unconventional but highly effective coaching technique. He always supported me and layered in new advice and strategies to try. My skills grew with each course that we tackled.

Onlookers thought we were professionals and were surprised to learn that we never kept score. In fact, we rarely shot the course as dictated. Correct etiquette required the shooter to enter the stand and observe the targets before shooting. The course card outlined how the targets were presented, typically either as a report pair pulled in series or a double pulled together. Russ never liked the formality, and he stepped into the stand and shot without ever seeing the targets.

"Birds don't announce where they're going to fly. They just fly," he said.

He typically slaughtered both targets without much effort, and then I had a license to mess with him. I pulled them before he was ready, pulled them out of order, pulled doubles, or whatever offered a challenge. When I stumped him, instead of getting frustrated, he looked back and flashed a glowing smile. He made shots I never saw another shooter make. Targets exploded seconds after leaving the trap, deep in the woods where I could barely see them, or in a rapid succession that seemed supernatural. I'd shake my head and lovingly tell him he was a jackass.

Even more impressive than his shooting was watching him make friends everywhere we went. I didn't consider myself shy by any means, but I liked to keep to myself or my group when presented with new people. Not Russ. He struck up a conversation with anyone, and within sixty seconds, they were laughing. On the sporting clays course, at a bar, at the gas station, it didn't matter. He sought eye contact and connection in a way that was foreign to me. Each new venue brought him at least one or two business cards from people who somehow wanted to connect with him.

My thirtieth birthday stands out. We were in Midland, Texas, and shot a range that seemed to be near only oil fields. It was in the middle of nowhere, and I thought we'd gotten lost. I kept saying, "This can't be right. This really can't be right," until suddenly, we saw the welcome sign.

The terrain was as flat and as hot as Texas could dish out, but they'd built forty-foot towers that housed the traps to make it interesting. We were sweaty, sticky, and covered with dust, but we smiled with each highflier, and adrenaline rushed as each target disintegrated into the blue sky.

After a full day of shooting, we settled into a hotel, cleaned up, and walked across the street to an Outback Steakhouse. If you had asked me at any point in my twenties if I thought I'd be spending the night of my thirtieth birthday in Midland, Texas, eating at an Outback, I'd have said you were crazy. But there we were, and we were having a blast. Russ made friends with everyone sitting at the bar. By the end of the evening, all the patrons were singing Happy Birthday and buying me drinks. I laughed so hard I had to run to the bathroom to keep from peeing my pants. We stumbled back to our hotel, and I felt happy. It was us, a truck, some supplies, and a two-star hotel—and I was utterly content.

That was Russ, the man I loved. Funny, charming, and amazingly smart. I wanted to keep that man with me as long as I could, even if it was only a memory.

* * *

After over twelve hours of travel, I finally made it to Sacramento. Kathy waited for me at the airport, patiently reading while my delayed itinerary caught up with hers. The slew of text messages from Russ stopped, and I vowed to ignore any drama for the weekend. My mother would handle it and let me know if she couldn't. I was there to enjoy Shannon's day and meet the woman who made my friend so happy.

I'd been to many weddings over the years. They were usually fun, but they also had their share of awkwardness. Second cousins crowded the much-argued guest list, venue changes shuttled people like well-dressed lemmings, and the happy couple flitted from table to table like misplaced diplomats.

But this wedding was different. The ceremony and reception were nestled in the backyard of Shannon and Rachel's friend's house. It had lush, soft-smelling gardens, a large pergola decorated with string lights, and a spa-like pool adding to the peaceful atmosphere. Kathy and I only knew Shannon's family. We didn't even know the other bride, but somehow, everyone made us feel right at home. We joined in on conversations and shared funny stories.

As Shannon and Rachel swapped their vows, the calm in their faces mesmerized me. They stared at each other, and I felt their love and the partnership they forged. Suddenly, all I could see was Russ's face in front of me. Those soft, telling eyes gazing into every part of me. His body wrapped around mine, covering me with warmth and comfort. A wave of happiness engulfed me, and I realized, as much as I was trying to remember him, it had been a long time since I *felt* him. Felt that moment of peace as he embraced me. Felt the aha as he planted a new idea in my head. Felt the security of knowing my partner was there for support. I fought back the tears, happy my friend found that kind of love but destroyed that I had lost mine.

After the ceremony, we melded back into conversation and laughter. Shannon's parents and sister were always dear to my heart and adopted me, if not in presence, then in spirit. We dug up our shared memories and laughed at old references that only we knew. Eventually, the inevitable question came. It was so simple, yet so complicated at the same time. "How's Russ?"

I could tell by the expressions on their faces that Shannon hadn't told them, which made perfect sense. She knew we weren't sharing with everyone, and she was a vault when it came to secrets. I could trust her with anything. I paused and thought through all the ways that I deflected the question so many times before. *He's fine . . . Oh, you know, Russ, still as crazy as ever . . . Doing well and keeping busy . . . As usual, hard to keep him out of trouble.* Most people asked only to make conversation. But Shannon's family had known me since I was nineteen years old. I couldn't be true to myself or them if I parroted a standard line of defense.

So, it all came out. The fighting, the loss, the confusion, the diagnosis. All of it. When I'd told others, I'd seen the shock and paralysis in their posture. The panic as they searched for words to make me feel better and make it all go away, knowing those words didn't exist. But Shannon's family listened and asked questions to understand. And when I started to break down, Harold, Shannon's father, came toward me and gave me a big Harold hug. His arms wrapped around me like a safe harbor in a storm. I sobbed, overwhelmed by sorrow but consoled in the comfort of his embrace. I realized that sometimes words weren't the best thing to offer someone.

Shannon and Rachel rejoined the wedding after their photo session. The DJ came alive, and before long, the whole group congregated on the dance floor. Shannon sought me out and pulled me aside.

"I'm so glad you're here. I know with everything going on, it couldn't have been easy to come."

I'd pulled myself back together after my Harold hug, but it was still fresh. "I wouldn't miss it. You know that."

"How are you doing? It must be so hard," she asked.

"Yeah, it is. But you don't want to hear about any of that on your wedding day. Today is about you, not me."

"I haven't seen you in so long, and catching up was one of the things I was looking forward to today." She paused, sensing my defenses. "I remember when you and Russ first started dating. How freaking happy you were and the way he looked at you. He was your person. Now that I have my person, I can imagine how hard it must be to watch him suffer."

I took a deep breath and avoided her probing eyes. But it didn't stop her.

"Cut the shit, Nicole. It's me. You don't have to be strong with me. Be strong for everyone else, but you don't have to be strong for me."

Like a guided missile, she unearthed my deepest torment. I was so freaking tired of being strong. I had to be strong for the kids, making them feel like everything was okay and normal. I had to be strong at work, leading everyone through each technical hurdle and challenge. I had to be strong to keep the house running, learning new things I'd never done before. And I had to be strong for the one person I relied upon. The person who gave me strength and grounded me in everything I did. But now, that person was slowly becoming more of a burden. He dragged me down into depths I'd never been before. So, I was forced to become stronger in order to survive. But I was so tired, tired of being strong.

I saw that my isolation was a partner to his illness. Fear and embarrassment swept in with the chaos that surrounded me. I struggled to keep his mental state hidden but hiding it was hiding me and who I was becoming. I needed Harold hugs and probing eyes and people to check in on me—not on Russ, but on *me*.

So, I sat there and cried with the bride. I unloaded not the facts but the *feelings*. I felt like the worst wedding guest in history, but I also experienced an enormous wave of relief.

Kathy was waiting for me as I came out of the bathroom to freshen up.

"Where the fuck have you been?"

I could tell she was beyond tipsy because the frequency of her curse words went up exponentially.

"I need a fucking partner on the fucking dance floor," she continued, "like right fucking now!" The smile on her face made me laugh and reminded me we were there to celebrate.

The rest of the evening was incredible. Kathy and I danced like two women on a Zumba retreat. Every song brought bigger and more ridiculous theatrics that channeled a younger, more carefree version of me. By the time the DJ played "Baby Got Back," we had recruited a dozen new friends, and all were in on the action.

In college, I always had the most fun when I was a little tipsy, but everyone else around me was drunk. Like a puppeteer pulling strings, I convinced my friends to perform ridiculous antics that became epic stories. It was a skill I'd learned from Shannon, and I was still her faithful padawan. So, when Kathy complained about how hot she was, I saw my opening.

"Why don't you go in the pool? That would feel amazing," I suggested.

"But I don't have a suit, silly," she protested as she stumbled a bit.

"Who cares? Everyone is a sweaty mess anyway. Go in your dress. With this low humidity, it'll dry fast."

Her face beamed with the possibility. After about five more minutes of cajoling, Kathy was thoroughly drenched. Then it was Shannon's sister, her mom, her dad, her niece—a half dozen people jumped in the pool in full-fledged wedding attire.

As I watched from a lounge chair, Shannon's niece called to me. "Nicole, this whole thing was your idea. Why aren't you in here?"

I looked at her soaked in her formal wear and said, "Eva, I want to give you a little chemistry lesson. I am what they call the catalyst. I *start* the chemical reaction, but I'm not *part* of the chemical reaction. I remain unchanged—and dry."

I shamelessly laughed at my nerdy joke and wished Russ was there to share the moment.

Kathy and I stayed until nearly 1:00 a.m., even though we had an early flight in the morning. I stole a moment with Rachel and thanked her for being stubborn enough to break through Shannon's protective shell. After all, Shannon and I got along so well because we were so much alike.

As I relived the weekend on the plane ride home, I stifled back tears. I hadn't felt like myself in so long. I used to be carefree and fun. Now, I was what everyone else needed, but I was losing myself in the process. The thought of home had once brought so much comfort, warmth, and support. But as I thought about going home, all I felt was dread.

7

Shit Happens

May 2017

Hypometabolism is severe in the inferior left parietal convexity and throughout the temporal lobes. As seen on the parasagittal images, metabolic activity is diminished in the cingulate gyrus and precuneus bilaterally, left greater than right. Despite the lack of cerebral atrophy (as seen on MR and CT), the degree of hypometabolism (as seen on PET) is compatible with advanced-stage disease. The pattern is most consistent with Alzheimer's Dementia.

I'd read the PET scan report nearly a dozen times in the last five months. I located pictures of the brain on Google and researched each lobe and its function as if figuring it out would unlock the mystery brewing inside my husband. In the end, only a few words resonated: *Alzheimer's dementia, advanced-stage disease.* The words repeated in my head even though the diagnosis didn't make sense.

Russ was only sixty-one. Yes, his dad had unspecified dementia, but he was in his late eighties, and he was eighty-nine when he died. Russ was fit, ate a Mediterranean diet, and had no comorbidities. There had to be another explanation for what was going on with him.

I researched other causes of dementia and asked the doctors to test him. They looked at me like I was crazy but must have figured it was easier to write the order than to argue. They tested his thyroid; his TSH was normal. They tested for syphilis and HIV—talk about not knowing which answer I was rooting for—and they were negative. They tested with the most extensive Alzheimer's genetic panel that I could find. APOE4, negative. APP, negative. PSEN1 and PSEN2, negative. He had *none* of the markers that predisposed him for Alzheimer's at such an early age. There *must* be another reason for his decline. I pleaded for other causes or reasons for his symptoms. I got nothing but a prescription for Aricept.

"Does it help?" I asked.

"It might for a little while," they answered. *What kind of answer is that? I'd fire an engineer that came to me with that kind of solution to a catastrophic problem.*

* * *

We were sitting in the lobby of our fourth neurologist. The doctors we'd visited before offered no insight, no answers to any of my questions. But Dr. Craven was the top dementia expert in the area. Two other doctors recommended him. My folder that contained Russ's lab results sat on my lap. It was nearly an inch thick, and the PET scan report was right on top. *The pattern is most consistent with Alzheimer's Dementia.* I reread those words, and they still didn't make sense.

Russ was fidgety and nervous. He was beginning to hate doctors, and every visit brought a series of repercussions. He yelled about how he didn't want to go, how they didn't help, and how they humiliated him with their questions. In the beginning, I argued with him with a genuine belief that we needed to go. We needed to figure this out. But after months of doctor after doctor with no straight answers, I was beginning to believe he might be right.

The blue folder in my lap was a formality since I already sent his lab work via fax. Working in medical devices, I heard about the wonders of

Electronic Health Records and how they would revolutionize patient care. Each time I listened to the "urrrr EEEE urrr NNNGGGG" of the fax machine, I wondered when this revolution would pull us out of the 1980s. I sent CDs containing the MRI and PET scan images before our visit. I wrote a four-page patient history of Russ's case and sent it over to Dr. Craven's assistant days ago. Actually, it was a three-page patient history because the fourth page was a list of questions for the doctor. I was prepared. Today was the day I would get answers.

The nurse did the standard workup of blood pressure, pulse, and weight and shuttled us into an examination room. A neurological fellow came in to do the initial assessment. At this point, I could almost administer it myself. What month is it? What state are we in? Draw a clock. Play tic-tac-toe. List all the animals you can think of. It was the standard dementia assessment playbook. Every time Russ got lost in a question, he became more and more frustrated.

I was relieved when Dr. Craven came in. Finally, we could get down to business. Although he asked some of the same questions as the fellow, he did it with a demeanor that put Russ at ease. When we got through his mandatory checklist, he turned and looked at me.

"So, what do we have here? Do you have his imaging results?"

My eyes indicated my confusion. "Yes, I sent the CDs over a week ago. I also sent all of his labs and a summary of his patient history."

"Hmm. Okay. Let me see if I can get my assistant to get those ready for me."

The same assistant I emailed twice and called four times? Wasn't she supposed to do that before the appointment? My years as an executive taught me to use the censorship chip that I installed between my brain and my mouth.

"I have everything here in my folder. I even have a copy of the imaging CD."

"Great. Let's take a look," Dr. Craven said as he inserted the disc into the computer. He then futzed around for ten minutes, trying to open the file, failing, futzing, and failing again. My anxiety grew as I sensed Russ getting antsy. When the doctor finally opened the file, he studied the images. We sat in silence. *Shit. Couldn't he have done this before the appointment? When I meet with someone, I prepare for the damn meeting. I don't walk in cold. And my meetings don't deal with life-and-death decisions like his do. This is ridiculous.*

Dr. Craven looked up from the PC.

"Well, based upon our discussion and some of his symptoms, I was worried he might have Frontal Temporal Dementia. But looking at the images, I agree that Alzheimer's is the right diagnosis."

Russ stood up. He couldn't take it anymore. "I have to take a piss," he said as he stormed out of the room.

When the door closed, I looked directly at the doctor. "Dr. Craven, I know what the PET scan says. What I don't understand is why. Russ is sixty-one, and he is declining so fast. I've been researching, and everything I find says it's rare to see Alzheimer's below the age of sixty-five if there isn't a genetic predisposition. And it's even rarer to see people with early-onset *and* rapid onset. He has no co-morbidities, he exercises, and he eats healthy. It doesn't make any sense. There has to be a reason this is happening."

He thumbed through the papers in my folder, but nothing grabbed his interest. He closed the folder, and we made eye contact.

"Well, Mrs. Bell, I know this isn't what you want to hear, but sometimes shit happens."

Those who know me know I'm pretty unflappable. My dad liked to tease; my older brother tortured me; I grew up in Boston. It was hard to ruffle my feathers. But in all my forty-one years, never had I wanted to strangle a man more than I wanted to strangle that doctor at that moment.

My mind raced. *Shit happens? Shit happens? Four years of medical school, three years of residency, three years of fellowship, decades in clinical practice, and the best you have to offer me is shit happens? Imagine if someone said that to me at work. Yeah, the robot isn't following any of our programming instructions, but you know, sometimes shit happens. No, shit doesn't happen. Shitstorm A causes shitstorm B and maybe rolls downhill to shitstorm C, but shit doesn't just fucking happen. Shit causes shit to happen, and it is your fucking job to figure out which shit caused this to happen to my husband!*

I sat there, paralyzed. My censorship chip had shorted, and I couldn't figure out how to make anything useful out of the tornado in my brain.

Before I could sort out my paralysis, Russ returned to the room. I wiped the look of shock off of my face and forced a smile.

Dr. Craven clicked through a few more images and then turned to face both of us. "So, you don't seem to think Aricept is helping. Have you tried Namenda?"

An automaton took over my body and asked, "Do you think it will help?"

"Well, it sometimes does. At least for a little while."

I shook my head. How anyone could live in this world of sometimes and little whiles was beyond me. I thought of the stakes. In maybe a year or two, my husband would lose everything: his knowledge, his skills, his memory, his continence, his dignity. And this was the best modern medicine had to offer? I forced back the tears. Once again, I had no answers, no root cause, and apparently, no hope.

* * *

I managed Russ's diagnosis exactly as I managed the challenges or problems I encountered at work; it was a problem, and I hadn't found the solution—yet. If I kept digging and probing in the right places, I would eventually figure it out. But with doctor after doctor providing no answers and no hope, I became lost. Every fiber of my being told me there had to be a reason, a root cause. Yes, shit happened, but that was getting hit by a truck or slipping on an icy sidewalk. This shit was a systematic deconstruction of my husband's brain, and there had to be a reason, or reasons, why. But the more I dug, the more I came up empty. Even worse, doctors chastised me for digging in the first place. He had Alzheimer's. Period. End of sentence. Actually, death sentence. I couldn't accept it, and yet, it kept staring me in the face.

Russ sensed my despair and attempted to refocus my energy. If this decline was inevitable, we needed to prepare. Our estate, our wills, our finances, they'd all been written before we had kids. We talked about changing everything and even sketched it out, but it never rose to the top of the list. Now, we needed to make sure the kids were taken care of no matter what happened. The thought made my stomach churn, but I knew he was right. It was amazing how the disease impacted parts of his brain so severely, while other parts could still think logically, soundly.

So, I immersed myself in preparations. Each phone call drove the message deeper into my brain. *My husband is dying.* I sorted through financial statements, tax documents, trust documents, every file more painful than the last. *I have to prepare because my husband is dying.* I used vacation time to meet estate attorneys. They drafted and redrafted. *Every scenario, every permutation of my husband dying.*

I judged myself each time we told a new person about Russ's diagnosis. *How did he get so bad? Why didn't I see the signs sooner? Why didn't I know?*

I watched as Russ interacted with people, and I saw what I hadn't noticed before. His quick wit usually customized a comeback or joke for the precise situation, but now, he relied on a set of familiar phrases. A list of questions or choices got an, "I don't care" or, "Whatever you think is best." A jovial memory with a friend would spur a laugh and, "Now, that was freaking funny" or, "I still can't believe we did that," but lacked details and context. A conversation on current events got, "Yeah, I saw that on the news . . ." with a dwindling tail at the end, so the other person picked up the next words. And my personal favorite was, "Well, I'm sure it's the government's fault," which worked in a surprising number of conversations, regardless of political affiliation.

Two dozen such phrases lodged themselves in his daily interactions and masked his illness. Most of the people we saw regularly still didn't know. Russ's compensation phrases kept the conversation going, kept them laughing, and before long, they moved on, no wiser to what he was facing. I realized how superficial many of our encounters were. How superficial my encounters must have been to let so much go unseen.

I kept pressing on. After all our financial affairs were in order, I started taking over Russ's tasks at the house. During many of our fights, Russ insisted that I didn't appreciate everything he took care of at home. As I took on his responsibilities, one by one, I realized he was right. I arranged for our friend Susan to pick up the kids after school and take them to their activities. I found a landscaper to take care of the yard and irrigation system. I developed a list of subcontractors to fix problems: an electrician, a plumber, a handyman. I found companies to power wash the driveway, clean the gutters, and more. Before I knew it, a Rolodex of a dozen people replaced the things Russ did without me noticing. Suddenly, it didn't matter that my list was as long as his; it only mattered that I hadn't seen and hadn't appreciated. He tried to tell me, and instead of listening, I argued, I justified.

At night, I laid in bed, exhausted. My mind raced back and forth between everything I had to do and everything I hadn't done. To-do list, guilt, to-do list, guilt. It was a never-ending loop of agony that reminded me of my new reality—one where I didn't have anyone to rely on. One where every action item was mine. One where I was losing my best counsel and friend. I pushed all the thoughts away and started my new sleep routine. I rolled over and put my arm around him. As he stirred and reached to hold my hand, I enjoyed his presence and warmth. *Deep breaths. Stare into the darkness of your eyelids. Deep breaths.* Eventually, I faded off to sleep.

Chaos

August 2017

Every morning, I called my mom on my way to work. It was a ritual. I got myself ready, got the kids ready, fed the dogs, shuttled everyone to the car, dropped off the kids at school and daycare, and called my mom. In the beginning, I didn't tell her about my problems with Russ. I commented here or there but overall avoided the topic. However, after she witnessed his Silver Alert firsthand, there was no reason to hold back. Our conversations became a daily check-in. It was a chance to vent, to make sense of the chaos. It wasn't enough to relieve the stress, but it was at least one person who knew what was going on in my world.

Because she was a loving Mimi, one of her daily questions was, "So, how are the kids doing?" It was a question I asked myself twenty times a day. It was only a month ago that I told Ryan that Dad was sick. I explained as best as I could that the way Dad acted was not the way Dad used to be. Dad wasn't well, and it was our job to take care of him. What a burden for a seven-year-old. How did his little brain even process that information? What long-term impact would it have? What did our world look like through his eyes?

But as I watched my newly seven and almost four-year-old, they seemed normal. Ryan was playing baseball on a real team for the first time and glowed with excitement before every practice and game. Hailey was prolific in her artwork and was the one person in the house who always gave me snuggles. Their top concerns were Legos that didn't fit, stuffed animals with ripped seams, icky vegetables at dinner, and fireflies that missed their open jars.

I worked hard to keep them sheltered from my burden. Activities and play dates were always at parks or other people's houses. Year-round sports kept us out and about. And at home, when Russ was in a bad mood, I shuttled them upstairs to play pirates of the bedroom or whisked them into our bedroom to watch their favorite TV show. I even hired a contractor to finish our basement. A gym, a big playroom, a nice bathroom—it would be an oasis where the three of us could play when all else seemed lost.

Life with Russ wasn't all bad. Some days, he engaged and reminded me that his fun factor far exceeded mine. He chased the kids around the house while his fingers and roar threatened to tickle them. He spontaneously started a pillow fight, leaving the kids squealing with laughter. Or he initiated an epic paper airplane contest to see who could make the longest flier from the second-floor catwalk. In those moments, the kids adored him. Life felt almost normal. But there were other days where depression and sadness ruled his psyche. In our moments alone, he talked about his solution to the problem. He still had access to his guns, and I wondered if he would do it. My gut told me no, but I based that on the man I knew, not the man he was.

The upheaval in my life was palpable, but somehow, I managed to keep it together. I added a review of my blessings to my sleep routine and took comfort in the biggest blessing of all—the kids. The kids were thriving. But over time, I realized that Ryan wasn't.

We were a month into second grade. Most kids hadn't even finished summer camp, but our year-round calendar meant that school started in mid-July. It was always awkward to be back in school so early, but when our three-week fall track out came in the calm and cool of September, I thanked the modified calendar for the distributed breaks. Ryan was already racking up behavior demerits in school. Nearly every day, I received notes from his teachers for talking out of turn, horseplay with friends, not being prepared for his lessons—the same repeating pattern.

I didn't know whether to be the stern disciplinarian or the understanding and probing mom. Sometimes, which one showed up was a crapshoot based upon my day at work or the roller coaster with Russ. But one night, while I was putting Ryan to bed, probing mom showed up.

"Ryan, I want to talk a bit instead of reading tonight. Is that okay?" I asked.

He pushed himself upright in his bed and looked a little confused. "I guess. About what?"

"Well, it seems like you're getting in a lot of trouble at school. More so than last year. Is something going on in your new class?"

He diverted his eyes to the blue trucks on his blanket and shrugged his shoulders as an answer.

"Do you like your new teacher? Are you getting along with her?"

"Yeah, Mrs. Goodman is great. I like her a lot. That isn't it at all." He looked at me, but his eyes returned to the blue trucks when he realized that he acknowledged a problem.

"Well then, what is it? What's going on?"

He started to cry, at first in little whimpers and then in full-fledged sobs. "I don't know, Mom. Second grade is so confusing. It's so much harder than first. They move you from class to class, and you always have to have the right supplies, and then they give you instructions, but I'm not sure what they mean. I never know what to do. I'm so stupid!"

His confusion and worry wrapped my stomach in knots. "Ryan, you are the most amazing little boy I've ever known, and you are most certainly *not* stupid. What do you think it is about the second grade that's so different from first?"

He answered as he gasped for air between his sobs. "I don't know! It seems like all the other kids know what to do, and it takes me a while to catch up. Then I'm always behind. And they make you sit there for *soooo* long! I hate school."

I grasped for words to calm or help him, but his despair felt like a black hole pulling me in. I swallowed hard to force down my tears.

"Well, Ryan, school isn't optional, so we have to work together to figure this out. Maybe I can talk to your teachers and see what we can put in place to help? We can review assignments for the week and make sure we understand expectations. I'm not sure what the solution is yet, but I know we can make it better. How about I reach out to Mrs. Goodman, and we come up with a plan?"

His breathing calmed, and he looked at me and nodded. I stroked his head, like my mom used to do when I was young. Then I suggested, "How about we read a little anyway? One Dr. Seuss book won't take too long, but don't pick Fox in Sox! I'm not sure my tongue can handle that one."

He laughed and jumped out of bed to grab Wacky Wednesday, his current favorite. He was almost ready to donate his Dr. Seuss books to Hailey, but the mere suggestion sparked a renewed interest, and we now read them nightly. The diversion calmed him, and within minutes, I walked downstairs in a daze from our conversation.

Instinctively, I looked for Russ to share the experience and figure out what to do. When I got downstairs, he was already asleep. The mayhem of bedtime was too much, and he retreated to the quiet of our bedroom. Once again, I was on my own. I sat on the couch and began my analysis.

Could the stress of his dad's illness be too much for him? I was reviewing my immunology studies from grad school, so I could better manage Russ's care. I knew that prolonged stress altered the effectiveness of cortisol and took the brakes off critical inflammatory pathways. Inflammation in the brain could cause behavioral issues. It was a definite contender.

But this isn't new; it's been going on for a long time. Ryan's behavioral issues started in preschool. Russ and I joked about him throwing temper tantrums at six months old. I knew he was somewhere on the spectrum for attention deficit disorder or ADD. My brother was diagnosed later in life, and my mom said Ryan was just like him, always on the go. The constant behavior demerits in kindergarten caused us to talk to our pediatrician about a formal ADD assessment. He gave us a questionnaire to fill out but noted they wouldn't treat him until he was severely struggling either socially or academically. Great. I couldn't wait for that. I'd read about natural remedies and put him on a good multivitamin and fish oil. He seemed to improve, but in hindsight, it was a tide that ebbed and flowed.

What can I do to help him? I combed through the options: email his teachers, check his assignments, develop lists, help him plan and prepare. Then I remembered a conversation from a birthday party over a year ago. I was socializing to get to know the other moms of the kids in Ryan's grade. A question that kept coming up was, "What do you do for work?" It turned out that one of the moms owned a center for functional neurology called Brain Balance. My inner geek was fascinated and kept asking questions. The center focused on ADD and autistic kids, analyzing their brains' strengths and weaknesses and developing a program tailored to improve their weak areas. I researched a bit afterward and found the concept fascinating, but it went by the wayside with my focus on Russ. *I'll reach out to Rebecca again to learn more.*

Comforted that at least there were a few moves to make, I started putting my developing plan into action. I sent an email to all of Ryan's teachers. I sent a message to Rebecca. I looked through his daily folder and his agenda for the week. I didn't know what to do about my husband, but I was determined to figure out what to do about my son.

About a week later, I met Rebecca for lunch. She was a beautiful woman with short blond hair and piercing blue eyes. But when I first met her, it was her background that impressed me, not her looks. She was a doctor of chiropractic medicine and had extensive post-graduate education in neurology, neuro-behavioral disorders, and childhood development. She didn't wear it on her sleeve, but a few questions and answers demonstrated that she knew her stuff.

It was a beautiful day for late August, so we opted to sit outside on the patio. I told her in my message that I was reaching out because of Ryan and that I wanted to pick her brain about what she did. As soon as we sat down, she let out a sheepish smile.

"I have a story to tell you, and I'm not sure how you'll respond," she said.

Her words piqued my interest. "Don't worry. There isn't much that can shock or surprise me these days." She didn't know about Russ, but she knew the general bedlam of motherhood.

"Well, as you know, my son, Austin, was in Ryan's class in kindergarten. One day, Austin came home from school and asked me for a business card. The request was odd, so I asked him why. He looked up at me and told me that there was this boy named Ryan in his class, and he thought I could help him." She paused to judge my reaction. "Out of the mouths of babes, huh?"

I chuckled. I agonized over Ryan's struggle, wondering if the root cause was his inherent biology or our crazy environment. Meanwhile, a five-year-old effectively diagnosed him years before our situation came to a head.

"Wow, what an astute little kid. It seems like he was a couple of years ahead of me. Hopefully, I'm finally catching up." I laughed to let her know that she hadn't offended me. Instead, her honesty made me happy I'd reached out.

"I adore Ryan," she said. "I see him all the time when I lunch parent, and he is such a funny, sweet, charming little kid. I was happy when you messaged me because I do think Brain Balance can help him."

"Great. Tell me how it works. And go slow so I can keep up," I said, smiling.

She grabbed a napkin and drew a pyramid with four horizontal lines through it. She then labeled each of the five sections from bottom to top: Primitive Reflexes, Sensory Motor Skills, Fine Motor Skills & Equilibrium, Visual & Auditory Processing, and Synchronization.

"Okay, so the brain develops by layering on new skills, just like the layers of a pyramid. There are the primitive reflexes you're born with, like the ability to grasp a finger, and then the rest you develop over time. First comes gross motor skills like throwing a ball, then fine motor skills like picking up a Cheerio. Eventually, you learn to do complex tasks like reading and writing or maybe even playing a musical instrument." She pointed to the pyramid and marched her way up as she talked, demonstrating the level of each skill.

"Each layer of the pyramid feeds into how we experience the world and learn. It fuels our executive functioning and decision-making.

If any piece is underdeveloped, the brain works harder to keep up. Imagine trying to build the top layer of the pyramid when the four layers below have missing pieces. It's going to be harder, right? In ADD kids, there are usually several weak spots. As a result, they struggle and use inefficient pathways to collect information. Our program finds and addresses the weak areas. Once we've done that, kids put pieces together more efficiently, and they thrive."

She then described how her center does a combination of physical, sensory, and visual exercises that strengthen the weak pathways until they are on par with age level. Food is also a huge focus. Our modern diet is inflammatory, and gut inflammation leads to brain inflammation. The program cuts out gluten, dairy, and other problematic foods to heal the gut and brain. In my research for Russ, I'd read multiple articles linking brain and gut health, and their approach fit my findings. She referenced studies of improvements in social behavior, academic performance, and confidence. I loved the science of it. Plus, it was a viable solution that didn't involve experimenting with pharmaceuticals on my little boy.

When our lunches finally arrived, we veered away from science and asked each other more personal questions. She asked about my husband. No one at Ryan's school knew about Russ. I thought about telling his teachers, but I barely knew them, and we hadn't even told many of our friends. But Rebecca was easy to talk to, and I wondered if her neurology experience could help in any way. So, I told her Russ was diagnosed with early-onset Alzheimer's, and in addition to managing an ADD kid, I was also managing that.

The look on her face was a look of genuine concern, not pity. It confirmed my choice to tell her, and so I went on.

"I worry that Ryan's symptoms are being made worse by the situation at home. I do my best to shelter him, but it's so hard."

"I'm sure it is. I can't comment specifically on Ryan, but it's pretty typical for kids to struggle around third grade. Ryan is in the accelerated classes, right?" I confirmed that he was. "So, he's doing a third-grade curriculum even though he's still in second. They start transitioning away from memorizing facts to using concepts to solve problems. A lot of ADD kids are right-brain weak but have strong left brains. The left brain handles facts and figures and does fine with the early-grade memorization tasks. But when you start switching to more complex problem solving and contextual reading questions, you need more right brain, and they have trouble keeping up." She paused. "I can't share names, but I will say that I've had several other parents from their class reach out to me this month, so he isn't alone."

I felt a wave of relief. It helped to think that we weren't the cause of Ryan's problems.

Rebecca continued, "As for Russ, I know a great functional neurologist who works with dementia patients. The exercises and techniques are similar to what we use with kids, but the focus is the declining brain rather than the developing brain. It can't cure, but it does improve the quality of life and function in some cases. I can pass along her info?"

"That would be great," I said with a sincere interest in one breath but nothing but doubt in the next. Russ was declining so quickly, and he hated doctors, hated assessments, and hated brain exercises. I flashed back to the day of his first cognitive assessment—all the anger, all the resentment. *Let's focus on my boy, and then we'll see about Russ.*

Rebecca gave me the step-by-step to get Ryan an assessment. I left the lunch with a few more action items, but I felt relieved to have a resource to help my son.

As I got back to the car, I checked my messages and found four voicemails from Russ. He couldn't find his keys, and his rancor escalated with each message. *Damn it. I haven't even got my head around one crisis, and the next one begins. When did life become a rolling sequence of chaos?*

I put the car in drive and called him on Bluetooth. *Fix the crisis with Russ, go to work, fix the crises there, go home, fix more crises, rinse, lather, repeat.* I took a deep breath and powered ahead.

9

Awakening

October - December 2017

It was our typical morning whirlwind. The kids were dragging more than usual, and by my seventieth reminder to grab their water bottles, shoes, jacket, or whatever, I felt harried. Russ was also in a bad mood. He cursed out the weed whacker and shoved it in my face in the middle of breakfast. I tried to get him to focus on something else, but he wasn't having it. After a few minutes on YouTube, I figured out how to fix the stuck line and load a new spool. Another day, another new skill.

Not to mention I was up at 4:00 a.m. reviewing work documents. The FDA recently cleared our robotic system. It was a humungous victory for the team and me since the FDA hadn't approved another robot for abdominal surgery in seventeen years. We worked nonstop to make it happen. But after a brief afternoon of celebration, it was time to prepare for launch and the mass of plans and documents that went with it. *Great. Not even 7:00 a.m., and it already feels like a full day.*

After I shuttled the kids off to school and daycare, I called my mom as usual. Right away, I could hear that something was wrong.

"Nikki, I talked to Scott last night. I think you should call him."

I didn't have a great relationship with my brother, so we hadn't talked in a while.

"Uh, okay. Is something wrong with him? Jodi? The kids? What's going on?"

She hesitated. "Well, it's better if you talk to him. It's about Jodi and what's going on with her, and it may be super important for Russ."

Her evasiveness left me confused and annoyed. I had a full day of meetings ahead of me. I didn't have time for games. If there was a problem, spit it out. I hung up and fumbled to find my brother's number.

Scott was six and a half years older than me, and we were never close. When he was a teenager, I was the snot-nosed little kid he loved to torment. He practiced karate on me, fed me dirty words to say in front of Mom, made me do his chores—typical big brother stuff. The worst was when he decided to hide under my bed and pretend he was a monster. He made deep, scary noises, rattled the metal bed frame, and banged on the wall, making death seem imminent. Somehow, I mustered the strength to make a run for it, scurry downstairs, and plead for my parents' help. I leaped off the bed, but as soon as my foot touched the floor, he grabbed it and pulled me into the abyss. I fought against him with all my might, convinced some horrible creature was going to eat me. Suddenly the light turned on, and my mom stood there with a look of pure shock. As I pointed to the mysterious creature under my bed, I saw Scott lying there, laughing. His braces gleamed in pure delight.

Little torments like that happened daily. I grew accustomed to it and eventually grew stronger. Then, when I was a budding teenager, he was gone. College, medical school, residency. He was off building his life, and I was left behind like an only child. I didn't miss his antics, but despite the torture, I always looked up to him. We spent time together on holidays and called each other every few months. We were both busy. I wondered if he'd even pick up.

He answered on the second ring. We exchanged the standard pleasantries, and I quickly got down to business. My meetings started at 8:00 a.m., and the distance to the office was closing fast.

"So, Mom said something's going on with Jodi?" I asked.

"Well, you know how she's been dealing with a lot of health issues lately?"

I knew but didn't know at the same time. Scott and Jodi shared bits and pieces along the way. She had years of hormonal problems that caused vaginal bleeding almost every day. Constantly menstruating for years—I couldn't imagine. Her gynecologist implanted an intrauterine device or IUD to make it better, but it only made things worse. To fix the problem once and for all, she had a hysterectomy. Doctors removed her uterus and cervix but not her ovaries. That was a little over a year ago, and her health had been a mess ever since. She suffered from chronic anemia, and no doctor could tell her why. She wasn't bleeding internally and had no signs of infection, but her iron and blood cell counts took forever to improve. The few times we did see her, she was fatigued and sensitive to sights and sounds. She described it as a terrible flu that never went away. It was now October, and I hadn't talked to Scott since Father's Day, so I didn't know her current status.

"Yeah, I know a little. Is she okay?" I asked.

"Sort of. We finally figured out the problem after seeing dozens of doctors. She has Lyme disease along with three other tick-borne coinfections."

"What? I know Lyme can cause weird symptoms, but how does that link to all her hormonal issues? And the hysterectomy?"

"Well, Lyme can evade the immune system for years, but there's generally still some immune response, some inflammation. Inflammation can include a host of toxins that damage brain tissue. In Jodi's case, it impacted her hypothalamus, which controls hormone production. There's a lot of literature out there linking hormonal imbalances to Lyme."

I wasn't sure what to say. It was a lot to take in. "So, is that why the hysterectomy didn't work? I mean, it stopped the bleeding, but she's been so sick since then."

"Yeah, that's the thing about Lyme. You can have it for a while and not know it. Then you have a traumatic event or illness, and your immune system can't keep it at bay anymore. It gets worse—way worse.

I think the surgery triggered her Lyme to flare, and she hasn't been the same since. She says that after the surgery, she woke up different."

"How is she now?"

"Nick, it's been bad. We haven't shared a lot, but she's struggling. She goes weeks at a time where she can't even get out of bed."

"Holy shit. What are you guys going to do? Is she going on antibiotics?"

"We found a doctor in D.C. He's treated thousands of patients and is well-known in the Lyme world. She's on an intense protocol, but it takes months, even years, to get better. It's going to be a long haul, but at least we feel like we're on the right path."

I sighed. "Wow. What karma gods did we piss off to make both of our spouses so sick? When did life get so freaking complicated?"

"That's one of the things I wanted to talk to you about." I could hear the hesitation in his voice. "I've been doing a lot of reading on Lyme. You know me when I get into something interesting . . ."

It was true; although Scott had ADD, he had the kind that included hyperfocus. When something grabbed him, he researched it to the ends of the earth. It was why he flailed around in high school and even college but thrived in medical school. He needed to find his place, but once he did, he found his inner rock star.

He went on, "Well, Lyme is a type of bacteria called a spirochete. Remember when you had Russ tested for syphilis because it leads to dementia? Well, syphilis is also a spirochete, and it's been shown that they cross the blood-brain barrier. There's a ton of research on neuroborreliosis. The bacteria causing Lyme is *Borrelia burgdorferi*, so neuroborreliosis is Lyme in the brain. It causes brain inflammation and leads to all sorts of neurodegenerative diseases. Case reports have reported Lyme in patients diagnosed with multiple sclerosis, Parkinson's, and even Alzheimer's. Whether it's misdiagnosis or causal is hotly debated, but the link is there."

"I know it's linked to brain fog and confusion, but linked to Alzheimer's?"

"Yeah, I was reading this paper about autopsy results from people with Alzheimer's. They found spirochetes embedded in the plaques that are the hallmarks of the disease. It definitely could be causal for some patients. Lyme seems to love neural tissue."

"But we tested him, and it came back negative," I said. "How can I prove that's his issue?"

"The tests used for Lyme are awful. The ELISA and western blot, the gold standards, they misdiagnose most of the time. Even in people *known* to have Lyme because they presented with the typical bullseye rash, they only test positive 60 percent of the time. That's ridiculous—it's barely better than a coin flip. Jodi tested negative on both. The problem is that *Borrelia* is good at evading the immune system. It changes the expression of surface proteins and hides in the extracellular matrix that surrounds cells. That's why people like Jodi can go for years without feeling sick. Then weird symptoms pop up, and they get misdiagnosed. Or they have a crisis, and it flares. Unfortunately, she had both."

He went on, "Think about it. If the bacteria are good at evading the immune system, you aren't going to get a robust antibody response. And what do westerns and ELISAs test for? Antibodies. No wonder the tests suck."

"So, how did she get diagnosed?" I asked.

"The Lyme doctor tested her with a different method. It looks for the DNA of the bacteria itself, not antibodies. And it looks at a urine sample. *Borrelia* tends to colonize in the bladder of animals, making it easier to detect in urine than in blood."

"So, it's a PCR-based test?" I knew all about Polymerase Chain Reaction from my time in diagnostics. It searched for a specific DNA target and then amplified it so an optical sensor could detect it.

"Yeah. You can order it online from labs that specialize in Lyme. I'll email you what you need. Keep in mind, you can still test negative and be infected. It's a matter of sensitivity. But Russ is so sick. If he has it, it probably will show up."

I paused to collect my thoughts. "Scott, do you think this could be it? The reason? I've never heard about the link between Alzheimer's and Lyme."

"Nick, I know it sounds crazy, but you wouldn't believe the amount of neuro involvement in this disease. One day I was talking to Jodi, and she couldn't remember the kids' names. Not some random kids, *our* kids! Then another time she was talking, and she couldn't find the words. She stared at me and said, 'You know that thing . . . under you . . . that you're sitting on.' I stared at her and said, 'You mean the chair?' She couldn't remember the word for chair. I couldn't believe it."

"Yeah, I've seen word-finding issues with Russ too. Yesterday he was trying to talk about his truck, but he said airplane instead. And he can *never* remember the kids' schedule even though it's the same every day."

"Jodi is the same way. She could always remember every little detail about the kids—teacher's names, friends, schedule, all of it. Now, she has to write everything down, or she gets confused and forgets." He paused. "Has Russ had any other symptoms besides cognitive symptoms?"

Immediately, I made the connection. "You know, he's had a ton of shoulder and knee pain lately. I asked the neurologist about it, but he brushed it off and said Russ was old and probably had arthritis. I should have put it together, but I'd already ruled out Lyme after all this time."

"It sounds related. Jodi's hips have been a mess. I'm telling you, Nick; you need to check it out."

He shared more stories, more research. He gave me names of scientists, websites, and papers to pull. I jotted them down, stunned, not sure what to make of it all. As I hung up the phone, I stared out the windshield. A glance at my dashboard clock revealed it was 8:30 a.m. I had been in the parking lot outside my office for thirty-five minutes. I was late, but I couldn't move.

Why didn't this call come six months ago? I needed it then. I finally accepted the madness. I stopped raging against the machine. There was no way I could help him.

Or was there?

Russ has advanced-stage Alzheimer's. Even the most progressive doctors are only having success with early-stage disease. No one can stop the fires once the whole forest is lit. Who am I to think that I can?

But what if Lyme truly is the cause? I've suspected it from the beginning, but his test said no. But everything Scott said makes perfect sense. I heard that Lyme tests were horrible when I was working in diagnostics. PCR testing is a much better approach. It's very specific and reliable as long as there is enough target. Curing an infection seems doable—much less daunting than treating a nebulous Alzheimer's fiasco. Or am I being naive?

The inner conflict consumed me. The leather seat pressed on my back, and I became aware that if it wasn't supporting me, I'd be lying on the ground, paralyzed. My breath shallowed and quickened as if the weight of the decision sat on my chest. It should be easy. Order the damn kit. But it was so much more than that. I was deciding if I wanted to bring hope back into my life. I had released it so reluctantly, so bitterly, but it was now gone. I wasn't sure I had the strength to bring it back and then lose it again.

Then his face flashed in front of me. This was Russ. This was the man I loved. Despite the awfulness of recent history, if I could get him back, I had to try. I couldn't live with myself if I didn't.

So, I peeled myself off the seat and stepped out of the car. My legs took a minute to stabilize as I walked into my office and settled into my desk. I booted up my laptop, and before I could change my mind, I opened Scott's email and ordered the kit. As I clicked the order button, I laughed at myself. *Well, here's to hoping.*

The kit arrived about a week later. Russ snarled when I gave him the sample collection cup but complied without a fuss. After all, it wasn't another blood draw or a trip to a doctor's office. Just piss in the damn cup. I did it about a thousand times when I was pregnant.

The company promised results in three to four weeks, so I tried to put the test out of my mind. I focused on the latest in Alzheimer's prevention. Reducing sugar intake emerged as a common theme. The most common genetic mutation increasing the risk of Alzheimer's, APOE4, seemed to interfere with the brain's ability to use insulin. As a result, papers and articles referred to Alzheimer's as Type 3 diabetes or diabetes of the brain. Russ didn't have this mutation, but reduced sugar intake slowed disease progression in multiple studies, even in patients without APOE4. Ryan's Brain Balance program also called for low sugar, so the whole family got a diet remodel. I already felt less moody.

And if sugar was bad, Russ's brain needed another fuel source. Evolution figured this out for us and provided ketones. I'd heard all about "keto" diets and being in a state of "ketosis," but I didn't understand what it meant. The liver breaks down fats into energy molecules known as ketone bodies. These ketones are the primary fuel source when carbohydrates are scarce, a regular occurrence in hunter-gatherer days. Now, carbs are everywhere, and sustaining ketosis takes work. After reading a couple of keto diet books, I wondered if it was even possible for Russ. I'd come home and find that he ate five apples—the keto equivalent of the Enola Gay. I could eliminate sugary snacks in the house, but eliminate apples? Seriously?

Then I read about exogenous ketones. Instead of relying on ketone production in the liver, we could take them orally to elevate blood levels. Mary Newport's work used medium-chain triglyceride (MCT) and coconut oil as sources of exogenous ketones. She found it improved cognitive function in her husband, who also had Alzheimer's. I decided to try it with Russ. I mixed MCTs in his coffee, cooked with coconut oil wherever I could, and bought keto bars loaded with MCTs. It made his stomach a little upset initially, but I eased up his levels and waited to see the results.

Then there were supplements. I tried everything I could find with decent science behind it. Fish oil, turmeric, huperzine-A, ginkgo, Co-Q10, Vitamin D. He had a smoothie and at least ten pills to take every morning. Sometimes, they went down without a fight, and sometimes, it took five or six tries before he swallowed them.

Our new routine seemed natural when the results finally came. It was a Friday afternoon. The first of December. I was sitting at my desk prepping for the following week when I saw the email pop up on my phone. The notification glared at me like a creepy clown at a carnival. Was it friend or foe? I didn't want to open it at work, but I had to know. As I clicked on the file, I took a deep breath. *Prepare yourself for both outcomes. You'll figure it out either way.*

I read the report. "The highlighted microbes were detected in the submitted sample." There were two, *Borrelia burgdorferi* and *Bartonella henselae*. My eyes stared at the bright yellow that surrounded the words. *Borrelia burgdorferi*—the bacteria that caused Lyme disease. *Bartonella henselae*—the bacteria that caused Bartonellosis, or Cat Scratch Fever. The colloquial name made it seem nonthreatening, but I knew from my reading about Jodi's diagnosis that this other tick-borne illness was a beast in and of itself.

I sat there staring, mesmerized by the yellow glow. Suddenly, a thought snapped me out of my daze. I logged into my personal drive and pulled up our earlier results. September 2016: Western blot negative for *Borrelia burgdorferi*. That was fifteen months ago. For fifteen months, I'd searched for answers that never came, and his brain continued to rot. For fifteen months, I could have been researching, treating, and helping. Instead, for fifteen months, I'd been flailing, losing, and giving up. Fifteen fucking months.

I wrapped up work and went to my car. As soon as it started up, I called Scott. When he answered, I said, "You were right. You were absolutely right."

The rest of the month was a total blur. We were preparing to launch the robot in the US, so yet again, my Christmas present from work was an insane December. After I put the kids to bed, I'd retreat to my office and research doctors in the area, methods of treatment, case reports—anything that could put me on the right path to help Russ. I made appointments and updated my folder with his patient history and labs.

Then, of course, there was Christmas. My parents were coming, and so was Russ's brother, Doug. After their dad's funeral and the disaster that ensued, I finally called Doug and told him about Russ. The two reconciled, and Doug planned to join us for Christmas, the first time since Hailey had been a month old. Then there were my two little elves who I didn't want to disappoint on Christmas morning. The presents, the decorations, that stupid Elf on the Shelf, the food shopping, the dinner preparations—all of it. I was beginning to wonder if there was holiday cheer for any mom out there or if it was one big rolling month of tortuous to-do lists.

And because all of that wasn't enough, on top of everything, we started having issues with our dog, Radar.

Radar was our first baby. Russ and I always wanted to get a dog, but life in apartments with constant travel seemed too complicated for a furry friend. Once we decided to settle in North Carolina and build the house, we took the plunge. Russ wanted to get a Rat Terrier. He'd owned a Jack Russell Terrier before, and he loved that damn dog. Russ described her as fun, feisty, and loyal. I joked that he talked more fondly about the dog than he did about his family. But Jack Russell Terriers were intense. It took nearly an hour of exercise a day to keep her calm. Rat Terriers were similar in looks, stature, and intelligence, but they had an off button. He thought the breed would be perfect for us.

I'd never had a dog before. My parents always wanted one, but my mom wanted a small dog like a Shih Tzu, and my dad wanted a big dog like a German Shepherd. Instead of compromising on a medium dog, we ended up with no dog. My brother and I begged, but still no dog. Scott eventually got fish, but we hardly considered that a victory.

So, when it was time to add to our family, I jumped in headfirst. I found a breeder about an hour away, and she had a new litter. One dog stood out since he was the only boy. We laughed as he trounced over and nipped at all his sisters. His body was all white, but he had the most beautiful brown and black mix on his head, with each color accentuating his features. We knew he was the dog for us. And because we also knew that his cute floppy ears would turn up into alert, probing dishes ready to turn at any sound or signal, Russ proposed that we name him Radar. A year later, we added another sweet puppy with a light brown head and a brown and white body. His name, of course, was Sonar.

Radar was now ten and wasn't the nippy puppy we took home ages ago. He was a few pounds overweight, mostly because Russ wouldn't stop feeding him from the table. I begged Russ to stop. I even asked the vet to shame him by giving the "overweight dogs have a higher incidence of cardiovascular disease" lecture. Three pounds didn't seem like a big deal until it was three pounds on what should be a fourteen-pound dog. But overall, Radar seemed okay. He was more sluggish and tired than usual, but I figured he was overweight and old. I'd never had a dog before, so I didn't know what to expect.

Then, in mid-December, we noticed he was licking his hindquarters a lot. A weird growth protruded from his fur a few inches from his tail. I took him to the vet to check it out, and they diagnosed it as a skin tag that had become infected. It was large, inflamed, and bothering him, so the vet recommended surgery to remove it.

So as his Christmas present, poor Radar sat on the couch sporting the colossal cone of shame. The cone sucks for all dogs, but for little dogs, it's terrible. Every time he climbed the steps to the back porch, we heard scurry, scurry, slam! The cone nicked the edge of steps and strangled the poor guy. I took it off out of pure pity, but he went straight to licking again, forcing me to put it back on.

Everyone came for the holiday as planned, and I ran around the house like a frenetic meth addict. All the work fell flat on my shoulders. Russ hated other people helping in the kitchen. He said they were too rough and slammed things around.

"Look at these chips on the granite! The scratches!" he yelled.

I conceded and agreed not to accept help from others, but that meant *he* had to help me. That worked for a while, but now, everyone was trained not to help, and Russ couldn't help like before. Cooking and cleaning up after seven people on my own became yet another reason the holiday season didn't bring much cheer. Ho, ho, fucking ho.

Christmas Eve was exhausting. I made a big dinner trying out all new recipes because none of our traditional family recipes worked with our new diet. Staying off gluten and dairy was critical. There was so much evidence linking them to inflammation. Also, we'd committed to being gluten and dairy-free for Ryan's Brain Balance program, and I didn't want to send him the message that they were off-limits unless it was a holiday. Off-limits was off-limits. So, I researched and found recipes that worked for us and wouldn't make people vomit. Everyone asked for seconds, so it seemed like a hit.

Then we opened presents. Tradition required that we open gifts from the family on Christmas Eve and gifts from Santa on Christmas morning. Ryan loved his new board games. Scrabble, Clue, Connect Four. Finally, games I enjoyed rather than seventeen rounds of Candyland. Hailey flipped through the colors of her unicorn table light and snuggled inside her mermaid tail blanket. They opened present after present, laughing as Papa attempted to guess their contents through his keen sense of smell.

Once the kids were in bed dreaming of sugar plums or whatever, I still had work to do. Our basement was completed right before the holiday, and Santa's sleigh had a new playhouse for Hailey and a scooter for Ryan. I wanted to assemble them in advance but never got around to it. Yet another Christmas Eve, I cursed out poorly written instructions. My engineering brain couldn't let it go.

"Clear and unambiguous! Instructions should be clear and unambiguous!" It was a message I tried to impress on my engineers but never seemed to find in my purchases.

By the time I plopped down on the couch, it was almost midnight. Doug and Russ were still up, but my parents had long gone to bed.

"You know, Radar doesn't look too good," Doug said to break the silence.

I looked over at the Little Bo Peep cone framing his head. "Yeah, he hasn't been eating lately either. I'm beginning to think maybe the anesthesia from surgery made him sick."

Russ chimed in, "I've been telling you; he hasn't been right for a while. Something is wrong with him."

He had been telling me that, but he had also been telling me that something was wrong with everything, so I'd gotten used to ignoring most of it.

"How old is he now? Ten?" Doug asked. "He doesn't look good for ten. He's been on the couch the whole time I've been here. Other than going to the bathroom, he doesn't move. He doesn't beg at the table, follow anyone around, nothing."

I knew he was worse after the surgery, but I kept hoping it would get better.

"I'll call the vet as soon as they reopen after the holiday. Hopefully, he'll be better tomorrow."

But he wasn't. Christmas Day, the kids were ecstatic with their new basement and toys, but Radar still wouldn't eat. The day after Christmas, he started vomiting. On the 27th, I took him to the vet first thing in the morning. They suggested an ultrasound to see if there was a blockage or something else to explain his symptoms. The vet called with the results around 3:00 p.m.

"Mrs. Bell, the ultrasound technician finished the scan, and I am afraid I have bad news."

Oh shit.

"Radar has a huge mass in his abdomen."

"Huge? What do you mean huge?" I breathed quickly. I could barely get the words out.

"It's about the size of a fist. It looks like it's overtaking Radar's adrenal glands, his kidneys, and even his liver. Also, it's putting pressure on his vena cava. I'm afraid it isn't operable."

The shock of the news made it hard to think. "Cancer?" I asked.

"Well, we won't know for sure unless we do a biopsy, but I'm afraid it looks that way."

"I don't get it. You cleared him for surgery a week ago. A week ago, you said he was healthy and fine. He just had a little skin tag. Now, you're telling me he has a cancerous tumor the size of a fist! He is a little dog. The size of a fist!"

"I know, but all of his blood work was normal, and the tumor is internal, so there were no outward signs. There's no way we could have known without an ultrasound. I'm so sorry."

My throat throbbed as tears filled my eyes. My voice cracked. "So, what do we do?"

"Well, you can take him home, and he may live another week or so. The pressure on his vena cava is impacting blood flow, so he isn't likely to improve. He will be like he was when you brought him in. Or, you can have him euthanized here. I know it's a big decision, so you can take some time to think about it."

Euthanized? Euthanized? A week ago, he was fine, and now, I have to decide if he should be euthanized?

His big black ears and brown nose filled my mind. "How is he? Is he okay?"

"Yes, he's comfortable. We put him on IV fluids and nutrients, so he's pretty alert and active. But that's because he's on the IV. If you brought him home, I wouldn't expect the same behavior. Think about it and let us know your decision."

I put down my cell phone and looked around the house. My parents and Doug were on their way home. Russ was riding his bike. The kids were with our neighbors, the Driscolls. It was the first time in weeks I was alone. I collapsed on the kitchen floor and cried.

What are you doing, Nicole? A fist. A fist! Your dog has a tumor the size of a fist, and you didn't know? You didn't notice? Russ kept saying he seemed off. Not as feisty, tired all the time. But you had a thousand other things to do, and you brushed it off. He was old. He was overweight. You blamed it on Russ for feeding him too much.

You brushed it off, just like you did Russ's symptoms—his drinking, anger, and depression. You came up with reasons why it was happening— his retirement, stress from the kids, not enough time for us. Justify. Justify. Justify. Well, none of it was justified! All of the stories you told yourself were wrong. And he's had Lyme, for who knows how long. You knew. You thought of Lyme right away. But he tested negative, and you gave up. Even though you knew the test was crap, you gave up. Now, it might be too late. It's certainly too late for Radar.

I wondered how my life got so off track that I didn't notice the things that mattered most. My sister-in-law, my husband, my dog—this was my family, the ones I loved most. They were suffering, and I didn't even know. I'd focused on all the wrong things.

Russ came home and saw the look on my face. He sat down next to me, and I told him the news. He put his arm around me, and the wave of sorrow hit again. It consumed both of us.

The next day the Driscolls watched the kids while Russ and I drove to the vet. They took us to a room way in the back. In all of our visits, I'd never seen this room. I never knew it existed. We waited, and they brought Radar in. He ran right over and jumped on our laps. His tail wagged, and he licked our faces. I was amazed. He seemed like a puppy again. His body was slim. I guess his lack of appetite made him lose more weight than I thought. He was quicker, peppier. *This is how he is supposed to be.*

We petted him, played with him, and hugged him. Every time Russ and I looked each other in the eyes, we couldn't hold back our emotions. We didn't want our time with him to end.

When the vet came back in to check on us, she asked if we needed more time. It didn't seem like the time we needed was available to us.

Then she asked if we wanted to stay or go. I looked at Russ. Panic flooded his face, and he shook his head. I wasn't sure I could do it either. I wanted my last memory of him to be happy. To remember petting him like he was a puppy.

We sat in the parking lot for over an hour. All I could think about was how fast his tail wagged. *Why didn't I notice his tail never wagged anymore?*

10

Undertow

January 2018

There we were again, in the waiting room of another doctor's office. Russ thumbed through a copy of *Guns and Ammo* magazine. I watched as his choice of reading and camouflaged shirt elicited a nasty look from a petite woman who was also waiting. I didn't care. I was relieved I didn't have to fight with him for three hours to get him in the car. He wanted to come to this appointment, which was a welcome change.

After we received Russ's positive Lyme results, I researched Lyme-literate doctors in the area. All search avenues led me back to Dr. Parker in Raleigh. He specialized in Lyme and worked closely with the same doctor Jodi saw in DC. When his name first popped up, I kicked myself. I'd seen his practice a year and a half earlier when I first took Russ to an integrative medicine practitioner. If I'd selected him back then, we would be in an entirely different situation. But I chose another doctor based upon the recommendation of a colleague. Looking back, I realized her office specialized in mold and not Lyme. We fell through the cracks, and the lost time from that one simple decision haunted me.

It was our second trip to the office. Our first visit took over three hours. The physician's assistant did the most extensive patient and family history that I could have imagined. She was interested in everything from birth to the present. Russ could only remember bits and pieces, so I did my best to fill in the blanks. Gallbladder removed in his twenties. Torn Achilles tendon at age forty-five. Hypertension diagnosis at age forty-six. I never realized I would be the keeper of all his history and stories. If only I had a notebook during all those late-night dinner conversations.

When we first met with Dr. Parker, he spent an hour with us. It was a refreshing change from our fifteen-minute neurology appointments. He probed areas of Russ's history, did a physical exam, answered our questions, and ordered a series of labs. Russ appreciated how he explained everything. For the first time, he believed a doctor was trying to help him instead of shoving him off with a useless prescription. So, when I told him it was time to go back and see his lab results, he seemed excited.

A medical assistant opened the door and called for Russ. When she saw him, she smiled ear to ear. In our first visit, Russ told jokes and cracked her up laughing—something she didn't get a lot of in an office focused on chronic illness. She immediately hugged him, and Russ went into full entertainment mode, pouring on the charm and flattery. He reintroduced me as his lovely wife and "the boss" and carried on the entire time she took his vitals. For a moment, it felt like a routine physical.

We moved into the examination room, and within a few minutes, Dr. Parker and his PA joined us. Dr. Parker pulled up Russ's lab results, and one by one, he went through them, focusing on the abnormal ones. It was like drinking through a fire hose.

- His ferritin was high. This could be from a chronic infection or from a hereditary condition that caused him to store too much iron. Follow-up testing would confirm.
- His copper levels were abnormally low. This could be a dietary deficiency, or it could indicate Wilson's disease. Again, follow-up testing would confirm.

- Urine organic acid testing and antibody testing indicated elevated yeast levels and unfavorable bacterial overgrowth. This could contribute to brain fog and should be treated before starting Lyme treatment.
- His PCR test was negative for *Babesia duncani*, another tick-borne infection, but antibody testing showed that he was positive. This coinfection could be a big issue in his case.
- Previous doctors didn't think much of his elevated heavy metals, but Dr. Parker said it could be central to his case. He wanted to perform a chelation challenge test to pull the metals out of the tissue and see how bad it was.
- His testosterone was low. This was bad for brain health.
- His immune system was suppressed. His white blood cell count was low. His C4a was high, indicating inflammation. His CD57, natural killer cells, were low.

I took notes, but my head was spinning. We'd spent the last year and a half with doctors, and everyone told us he was normal. Normal, that is, except for his Alzheimer's. Now, we had lab after lab that showed issue after issue. Each result potentially worsened his dementia and indicated that an infection brewed. I didn't know whether to be relieved or angry. I looked over at Russ and saw nothing but confusion. He looked to me to sort it all out, but I was overwhelmed. The doctor did his best to explain, but the undertow pulled me, drowned me.

Dr. Parker must have sensed my distress because he stopped discussing the litany of lab results.

"Look, I know it's a lot. We run a series of labs to see what we are up against. Lyme rarely comes alone. Typically, when it's bad, other infections flare, hormones and nutrients get off balance, and the immune system is in the tank. The good news is, I now have a pretty good picture of what's going on."

"So, where do we go from here?" I asked.

"We need to start with his gut. The yeast and bacterial overgrowth are a big deal, and I can't start him on an aggressive antibiotic protocol for Lyme and coinfections if his gut is a mess. We'll do a thirty-day treatment for that, including diet changes, probiotics, and a course of antifungals and antibiotics. Then we'll check in and see if he's ready to start treatment for Lyme."

"And what does that involve?"

"We'll put him on a broad-spectrum course of antibiotics. You've probably heard that you can treat Lyme with two to four weeks of doxycycline. That treats the active spirochete form of the bacteria well, eliminating about 90 percent of them. The problem is that the bacteria also takes on atypical forms known as persister cells. Think of persister cells as a protection mechanism. When there are adverse conditions, like your immune response or antibiotics, the bacteria transform to protect themselves. It reduces its activity and rolls up into a tight ball that is much more resistant to antibiotics."

I glanced over at Russ. He looked numb.

Dr. Parker went on. "And that's not the only defense that they have. They also hide in biofilms, forming communities surrounded by a viscous, protective gum. The longer the infection lasts, the more persister cells and biofilms emerge. That's why doxycycline can be successful for an early-stage infection but isn't sufficient for chronic infections. We use a host of antibiotics to target the bacteria throughout the body and herbs to break up the biofilms. You'll also get some coverage for *Bartonella* and *Babesia* with the regimen, but we'll change up the meds later to address those specifically."

"And what about the blood-brain barrier?" I asked. "Will the antibiotics penetrate and treat the neuroborreliosis?"

"Well, for that, we'll want to put him on IV antibiotics, which has the best results for blood-brain barrier penetration. That means he'll need a PICC line—a peripherally inserted central catheter. That will allow you to give him the IVs at home since it will be three days a week. Plus, I'll also want him on other IVs for detox."

The undertow pulled me deeper out to sea. *I'm going to be administering IVs? I'm a pretty good wife and mom, but Florence Nightingale, I'm not.*

Dr. Parker saw my panic. "Don't worry. You don't have to know all of this now. We'll start with his gut and go from there. I'll also give you some reading material so you can familiarize yourself with what we are doing now and what's coming up ahead."

So many questions ran through my head, I wasn't sure what to ask next. The only question that mattered bubbled to the top.

"So, do you think it will work? Will he get better?"

"The thing about chronic Lyme is that it gets worse before it gets better. When you treat with antibiotics, lots of spirochetes die, and their bodies fragment. Toxins are released, and cellular debris is everywhere. It's like a garbage dump that your immune system needs to clean up. But there's so much of it, and his immune system is suppressed, so it won't be able to keep up. The buildup of waste leads to inflammation and a host of symptoms like fever, chills, and headache. We call them Herxheimer reactions, named after the researcher who first described the condition. We'll do all we can to detox and boost his immune function, but it can get worse before it gets better. It took him a while to get this sick, so it will take a while to get well."

"Like how long?" I asked.

"For most people, it can take eighteen to twenty-four months," he responded.

"Two years?" It was the first thing Russ said since our round of hellos. "Two years of this shit?"

"Yes," Dr. Parker replied. "It can get better as you go along, but this isn't a short process. We pulse the antibiotics to draw out the persister cells systematically. They can go dormant for a year or more, so you have to be vigilant, or you'll relapse."

Russ got restless, and I could tell our time was limited. I shifted the conversation to the treatment protocol for the coming month. Dr. Parker recommended two different detoxification products, one for the extracellular matrix and one for the liver. He recommended binders to start grabbing and expelling heavy metals. Until the PICC line was in place, we could come to the office and get IVs of glutathione, a powerful antioxidant and detoxifier, especially for the brain. He prescribed antifungals, antibiotics, and probiotics for his gut and phlebotomy blood draws to bring his ferritin levels down. He upped our dose of fish oil to promote immune clearance and brain health. I walked out with a packet of information and a slowly budding headache.

On the drive home, it was silent. I was overwhelmed. Leading a team of over fifty engineers, I was often in over my head. I managed people designing software and circuits, areas where I had little technical training. Despite that, I made my way through. I knew the basics, the lingo. I sensed the tension in a particular statement and pulled a loose thread. Fake it 'til you make it, I joked. But this was different. I didn't know when to push back. I had to take everything at face value. I'd been doing that for over eighteen months, and it hadn't served us well. It seemed like this was the right path, but how did I know? I really, really hated not knowing.

Over the next couple of weeks, I poured every spare moment into research. Of course, I started where everyone starts: the Internet. I quickly realized what I already knew. The Internet was a dangerous place to get information. My searches left me more confused than when I started.

Half of the articles insisted that chronic Lyme didn't exist. The Centers for Disease Control and Prevention, the CDC, claimed Lyme could be treated with two to four weeks of antibiotics. After that, anyone still sick didn't have chronic Lyme; they had Post-Treatment Lyme Disease Syndrome or PTLDS. But the causes of PTLDS were unknown. It could be an autoimmune response triggered by the bacteria. It could be a persistent but difficult to detect infection. It could be other issues unrelated to Lyme. As I read their position over and over again, it didn't make sense. One of their explanations for PTLDS was a "persistent but difficult to detect infection." Um, okay. Why couldn't that be Lyme?

The other half of the articles blamed Lyme for nearly every chronic disease on the planet: fibromyalgia, arthritis, chronic fatigue syndrome, multiple sclerosis, myocarditis, Parkinson's, Alzheimer's, scleroderma, depression, schizophrenia. The bacteria was invading our immune system and wreaking havoc. It infected joints, brain tissue, and cardiac tissue. It triggered autoimmune conditions, dementia, and mental illness. The disease was way under-reported and globally prevalent, not only in the American Northeast.

So, what to believe? Frustrated, I turned away from Internet articles and turned toward scientific articles on PubMed. The messages there were equally mixed. I scanned through titles and abstracts. For each article I found supporting chronic Lyme's existence, I found another attempting to debunk it. Clearly, I needed to read the articles to form my opinion, so I dug in. I found observational studies with no controls, failed attempts to reproduce past results, citations to other papers that didn't say what was claimed. The more I read, the more frustrated I became.

I had long been a steward of science. "In God we trust; all others must bring data." The quote from W. Edwards Deming was frequently touted at the FDA and always made me smile. I agreed. Data was pure. Data had no agenda. Data was just data.

But my career taught me this wasn't true. Data collected was only as good as the methods used. Science used mice and cell cultures that may not represent the complexity of a human. Researchers interpreted the data, and often their bias skewed the results. I'd seen engineers interpret the same results in opposite ways. Plus, people made mistakes. I once struggled for over a month with an experiment, having no idea why the results didn't match the theory. Then, I spent the day with my technician and realized that every time I instructed her to do a step for a minute and a half, she entered one minute and fifty seconds into the machine, completely trashing my analysis. Data wasn't always pure. It could be flawed.

I saw this debate raging in the medical community, and I didn't know whether to feel vindicated for finally finding my answers or crazy for believing in something so clearly outside mainstream medicine. Organizations like the CDC and the Infectious Disease Society of America should know what they are talking about, right?

On the other hand, mainstream thinking always evolves, even in science. If it didn't, we would still think the world was flat or that lobotomies were the best way to treat mental illness. No one believed that the bacteria H. pylori caused stomach ulcers, so Dr. Barry Marshall infected himself to prove it. Nutritional guidelines in the 1980s told us a low-fat diet was best. Now, leading experts tout that a high-fat, ketogenic diet is better for overall health. I needed to navigate a complex infectious disease, and I couldn't get a straight answer on eggs. Good for me? Bad for me? Different doctors, different answers. Argh! I was in the middle of a debate where my husband's life hung in the balance. I had the desire to learn and the skills to understand, but I was more lost than ever.

In engineering, we were taught never to believe in an experiment where the number of samples, "n," equaled 1. Strength came in numbers, and real science was repeatable. But science was failing me, and an "n" of 1 was how things got started. So, I turned to medical case reports.

Patient: seventy-six-year-old female. Progressive cognitive decline over the last twelve months, loss of weight, gait disturbance, and tremor. Diagnosed with neuroborreliosis after antibodies found in spinal fluid. Treated with antibiotics and recovered to age-appropriate cognitive performance. Currently, eighty-two years old and no gait or cognitive impairment.

Patient: seventy-one-year-old female. Admitted to the psychiatric department due to rapidly progressing dementia or delirium. Suspected Lyme due to history of tick bite and widespread rash. Treated with antibiotics, and cognitive performance improved. Patient stable five years post-treatment.

I found case after case. Some doctors treated with shorter stints of antibiotics, some longer, some with IVs, others with oral. I thought of Russ. His do nothing prognosis was bleak. I had to try. I talked to him about it repeatedly. What did he want? Was he up for the fight? Some days, he said he was, and others, he said he wasn't. I struggled to be his proxy, but I wanted him to be here, for me, for the kids. And he must have wanted to be here too because, after almost a year of a crushing diagnosis and countless threats to kill himself, he was still with us.

My training as an executive prepared me for this. I always preferred to make decisions logically, with data. But business and life didn't always work that way. I needed to move forward with considerable gaps in my information. So, I did what I do at work. I broke it down into the questions I needed to answer now, not next month, but right now.

The first question was whether I believed that Lyme was the cause of Russ's issues. The facts. He was a hunter. He was always in the woods. He'd lived in New Jersey, New Hampshire, North Carolina, areas known to be endemic with Lyme. I'd pulled dozens of ticks off of him. Alzheimer's didn't make sense. He had no co-morbidities. No family history. He was so young. He was declining so quickly. His illness started as only cognitive, but he developed a host of physical symptoms. He couldn't put on a shirt by himself because his shoulders hurt. He limped because of swelling and pain in his knee. That sounded like Lyme, even if the cognitive link was controversial. Finally, I had a positive PCR test result showing that the bacteria was in his body. It wasn't the CDC gold standard test, but it was the same method that detected hundreds of infectious diseases, including the flu. The science was there. Did I believe it was Lyme? Yes. The answer was yes.

The second question was if we should treat with antibiotics or with other methods. This one was trickier and more nuanced. I read about alternative therapeutic methods: herbals, immune modulation, homeopathics, even whole-body hyperthermia treatments. But the papers of successful case reports were all from antibiotics. Lyme was a bacterial infection. It made sense. The broad-spectrum approach would ensure if bacteria were there, they were dead. I wasn't sold on needing it for two years, but I didn't have to be right now. I needed to get started, and every day would bring more data. Should we treat with antibiotics? Again, the answer was yes.

I looked through the materials from Dr. Parker, and it was clear that treatment would be intense. This process wasn't something I could do on the side. I needed to be all in to help Russ and to get him through the series of pills, IVs, and adverse reactions. I needed to be focused, present. I couldn't miss the signs as I had for years. I needed more time to understand the research, the treatment. Something had to change.

By the end of January, I reached a decision. I needed to step back at work. I sat down with my boss and shared my situation. He knew bits and pieces, but it was time to fill him in on the rest. We worked out a plan where I could work half time, and the time I did work would be mostly from home. As I walked out of his office, I felt an enormous load lifted off my shoulders. Our Lyme treatment journey was about to begin. I was nervous, overwhelmed, and tired, but hopeful.

11

Treatment

March - April 2018

All day, I stared at the same bucket of pills.

Three weeks earlier, I met with Dr. Parker to go over Russ's plan for his second cycle of treatment and his first cycle of antibiotics. It was intense. He was on *eight* different antibiotics, each day with a different sequence of pills. Some three days a week, some four days a week, some five days a week. Then there was an anti-fungal twice a week to keep his yeast from propagating. And that was only the prescription medications.

Then there were the supplements. N-Acetyl Cysteine to raise his glutathione levels, a powerful antioxidant. Chlorella, cilantro, and seaweed to help with metal detoxification. Probiotics and L-glutamine to help his gut. Phosphatidyl Choline, omega fatty acids, and Burbur/Pinella to support brain function and perfusion. Turmeric to lower inflammation. Hawthorne to lower his blood pressure. A multi-vitamin and multi-mineral. I researched and learned about each one—what they did and who made the best products. I reached out to my brother, Scott, to take advantage of his physician discount where I could. We swapped pill stories: what our spouses were on and what seemed to be working.

Every Saturday was pill-sorting day. Hundreds of little pills carefully placed into fourteen containers, two for each day, AM and PM. It was too much to do in real time, so I pulled out the medication matrix and did it all in one fell swoop. I couldn't find a pillbox large enough to fit his cavalry of pills, so I improvised. I went on Amazon and purchased those plastic cups used as to-go containers for ketchup—or Jell-o shots in my wilder times. I labeled each container with a sharpie. Then, at the appointed time, I found the appropriate little bucket for that day and time. It was like my grandmother's pillbox on steroids.

In the morning, I put the pill bucket on the counter before dropping the kids at school.

"Here you go, babe. These are the pills for the morning. Please take them, and I'll make breakfast when I get back." I kissed Russ, and he nodded.

I shuttled the kids to the car and dropped them off in morning carpool. When I got back, the pills were still there.

"Russ, you didn't take your pills yet. We started the new antibiotic protocol, and it's super important. I know the first week was rough, but you're so much better. We need to stick with it."

It was true. The first week was hard. He was confused, tired, and some conversations were completely incomprehensible. But around day eight, he woke up with no pain. His mood improved. His cognitive function was still lacking, but it was better than it had been. It felt like a much-needed lifeline. It gave me confidence that we were on the right path. But only if he kept taking the damn pills.

He looked over at the counter and nodded. "Okay, I'll take them."

I felt a nudge and realized our new puppy was at my feet. His sweet little eyes looked up at me and made me smile. He was my grieving puppy. Within a week of losing Radar, I was on the Internet looking for breeders. I found a beautiful Rat Terrier that was due to have puppies in January, and before I knew it, I was filling out paperwork.

Junior, short for Radar Junior, had been with us about a week, and the kids were in love with his expressive brown face and soft little brown and white body. I loved him too, but I'd forgotten the work associated with a puppy. I thought our fenced-in backyard would make it easier than when we raised our first two dogs in an apartment. I could put him outside, and he would follow Sonar and go pee. No such luck. I looked past him and saw a tiny little pee stain on the living room rug. *Why on Earth did I get a puppy in the middle of this?*

I put the dogs outside, cleaned up the mess, grabbed a snack, and went up to my office to work. Back-to-back conference calls kept me busy through lunch, so it was about 3:00 when I made it back downstairs. When I wasn't working, I usually researched treatments or spent time with Russ. But this afternoon, I had a hair appointment at 3:30. Silly as it was, getting my hair done was the only thing that I did for myself. The kids or Russ consumed everything else. It was a coveted three hours every six weeks. Pathetic, but reality.

As I rushed through the kitchen, I saw that the pills were gone. I breathed a sigh of relief. *Finally.* I went to find Russ to tell him my plans. He was in his office staring at his computer. In front of him lay the bucket of pills, still full. He moved them, but he didn't take them. This time I got snippy.

"Russ, your AM pills are becoming your PM pills. You need to take them, or you're going to get worse."

My frustration triggered him. "Do you see how many pills are in this freaking thing? It's ridiculous! How do you know they even help?"

"You're already better than you were a few weeks ago, and they won't help if you don't take them." I looked at my watch. "Look, I have to go. If I miss this appointment, I won't be able to go for weeks. Please take the damn pills! I'll see you when I get back."

After my haircut, I stopped at Panera to pick up some salads for dinner. The kids were with our new afternoon sitter, Pauline, until about 8:00 p.m. It was something we started doing once a week, so I could run errands or have a quiet evening with Russ. No cooking. No screaming and fighting at dinnertime. No drama. It was a much-needed break.

When I got home, I felt pretty good about myself. My grays were gone, my hair looked great, and I had dinner in my hands.

I hung my purse in the cubbies by the garage and looked around for Russ. When I turned the corner to the kitchen, I saw them, back in their rightful place on the counter, the same damn bucket of pills. At this point, they taunted me.

We ate dinner in silence. I didn't know what to say. I wanted to scream. We were two months into treatment, and this argument was like a bad mixtape on repeat. Dozens of replays but still no understanding. No resolution. An infinite loop, each repetition more grating than the last.

When we finished dinner, he asked, "So, are you mad at me?"

I took a deep breath and tried to figure out how to respond. After a moment, I said, "I'm not mad. I'm lost. I've spent weeks getting us to this point, getting us to that bucket of pills. And it seems to be working. You're feeling better. You can raise your arms above your head for the first time in months. You look better. But it feels like every day, twice a day, it's the same fight. I have to nag you more than I do the kids. Frankly, it's exhausting."

"What if I don't want to fight? I've had a good life. I've got nothing to live for."

The look of apathy in his eyes churned my emotions. Pains throbbed in my head, throat, and gut. I stared at him, trying to elicit something, but I saw only emptiness.

"You know the people I live for every day are right in this house: you, the kids, even the damn dogs. Every day, I give and I fight because I love you and them with all my heart. And for you to sit here and say you have nothing and throw away the chance to be with us—and see our amazing kids grow up—it makes me want to throw up. I don't know if it's the sickness talking or you, but it's bullshit. And it hurts. A lot."

"Well, that's it then. I'll leave tomorrow."

There it was again, the mythical escape. Sometimes, it was a nonexistent job opportunity in California. Sometimes, it was heading back home to Atlanta. I laughed at that one since everyone was gone except for his brother Doug, and there was no way in hell Doug would take care of him.

"That's right. Leave. Go to Atlanta. You'll end up in jail or worse."

"I don't care." His voice was monotonous, lifeless.

"I can't have this argument again. I just can't. If you don't want to fight, then don't. But don't keep changing your mind because it's torturing me."

I left the room. The logic and passion were gone, maybe forever. I hoped not, but I worried more about it every day. I went into the bedroom and took a long, hot shower. The damn pills ruined my evening, so why not ruin my salon hair along with it.

I came out right before the kids got home. *Time to put my game face on and pretend everything is normal. Whatever that means.*

I walked into the kitchen and saw the bucket—it was empty. *I guess we fight, at least for one more day.*

* * *

The first round of antibiotics was for six weeks. By week four, Russ was doing well. He put on his shirt without cursing. He rode his bike and power washed the driveway. His mood improved. The constant battle over pills stopped, and he popped them down whenever I put them out. For the first time in a while, I felt hope. Maybe my future could be the life I thought it would. Maybe my kids could have a father.

But bacteria have been evolving for billions of years. They're experts at self-preservation. When exposed to hostile environments, like antibiotics, they go dormant or become resistant. The bacteria causing Lyme, *Borrelia burgdorferi*, develops persister cells that become inactive. Waiting. Later, when conditions are favorable, they reemerge and wreak havoc.

Borrelia also forms close-knit bacterial communities similar to our cities. They fill and surround the city with a viscous biofilm that protects the community and provides nutrients. Studies in cell cultures show that biofilms make bacteria orders of magnitude less susceptible to antibiotics. Antibiotics may even trigger the bacteria to produce more biofilm, making the barrier stronger and increasing the ability to evade treatment.

In Russ's protocol, we had a two-week break between every six-week cycle of antibiotics. This "pulsing" of medication encouraged dormant bacteria to reemerge, making them susceptible to the next round of treatment. Dr. Parker warned that patients often felt awful during these two weeks. Symptoms returned, many times worse than before. People craved the antibiotics, consciously or subconsciously longing for the medicine that killed off the bugs and the pain.

I'd also read several articles questioning whether persister cells and biofilms were relevant to Lyme. Scientists observed them in cell cultures but questioned their existence in humans. If they didn't form inside the body, then it seemed logical that one round of antibiotics would be sufficient, precisely as the CDC said. So, I waited to see what would happen with Russ.

Our first two weeks off was as the doctor warned—hell on Earth.

It started with fatigue. Russ napped for vast portions of the day or went to bed for the night by 4:00 p.m. Then his pains returned. His arms, knees, and back throbbed with aches. Next, confusion set in. He put his keys in the safe, but fifteen minutes later, he forgot where they were and was frantic. He lost his flashlight. He couldn't turn on the power washer. Every thirty minutes, it was something new.

I spent the entire week on defense. When he was awake, he required constant attention. Lost items were a recurrent theme, so I put Bluetooth trackers on all his daily essentials.

"You can't find it? Let me check my app. Oh, here it is. No need to worry."

I figured out how to fix and run the power washer. That was something new—go me, girl power. We occupied ourselves with long walks, rides in the car, errands. I kept things under control, but every day, I grew more and more tired.

When he went back on antibiotics, the first week was still rough. Around day eight, his pain went away, but his mood was unstable. He was fine most of the day, and then there'd be a trigger. It could be me asking him to take his pills. It could be the kids laughing too loud. It could be our neighbor flinging rocks with a lawnmower. It could be anything. He turned nasty for an hour or more. Yelling, ranting, belittling. Then, the hammer uncocked, and he became conciliatory and pleasant.

This was Russ's unstable state when it was time to get his PICC line placed. Peripherally inserted central catheter—I had no idea how it worked, so I Googled images. One end of a thin, soft tube would dangle from his arm to allow easy access for IVs and blood draws. The other end of the tube would rest in a larger vein leading to his heart. With the PICC line in place, I could administer IV antibiotics at home three times a week. IV antibiotics penetrated the blood-brain barrier, a selective wall protecting access to Russ's top battleground, his brain. I still wasn't wild about giving IVs, but I wanted to slaughter every last little bug stealing my husband.

I talked to Russ for weeks about the PICC line and the IV treatments. I explained everything as best as I could: the whats, the whys, the hows, the whens. I wanted him to be prepared. But I forgot I wasn't talking to Russ. I was talking to a shell that looked like Russ.

On the day of the surgery, he was confused.

"What are we doing? Where are we going? Who is this doctor?"

He repeated the same questions again and again. I grew nervous. If I couldn't get him to swallow a bucket of pills, how in the world was I going to get him to have surgery?

The fact that there was new ownership of the vascular surgery center added to the confusion. A large hospital system acquired the office, and mayhem resulted. The computer system was new; the nursing staff was new; supplies were in unknown places; the office manager didn't work on Fridays. The disorganized mess fueled Russ's growing anxiety. His eyes glared at me like lasers, ready to cut me in half at the next complication or delay.

Somehow, we got through it. Afterward, Russ said the doctor was rough and that it hurt like hell. I didn't give it much credence because he was cranky and tended to exaggerate. Plus, it was time for lunch, and we were both starving.

We grabbed a bite to eat and headed to Dr. Parker's office. Our favorite nurse, Ashley, walked me through how to administer an IV and care for the PICC line. I left with a shopping bag full of supplies and a binder of instructions and notes. It seemed simple, but my nerves still twitched. There was a damn good reason I was an engineer and not a nurse. I could manage a design review for a surgical robot, but the thought of flushing saline through my husband's veins made me queasy.

As we drove home, the tube that stuck out of Russ's arm dominated my thoughts. I wasn't prepared for the day-to-day challenges ahead. How would I give him treatments? Ashley wrapped the PICC line in an adhesive wrap, and it was a pain to undo. How would he shower? It had to stay dry, or it could get infected. Where would I hang the IV bag? I didn't have a pole like they did in the doctor's office.

When we got home, I logged into Amazon. I ordered a PICC sleeve for his arm to support the tubing and keep his arm comfortable. It folded down to administer treatments and would be more comfortable than the wrap. I ordered shower sleeves to keep it dry when he bathed. Finally, I ordered a simple IV pole to hold his bags during treatment. *You can do this, Nicole. You can do this.*

On Sunday morning, it was time for our first home IV. The responsibility hovered around me like a horsefly, right there, no matter how many times I shooed it away. The kids went downstairs to watch a movie, and I knew it was time. I asked Russ if he was ready, even if I wasn't. He responded, "I guess so," which I took as a good sign. But once again, I forgot that a stand-in answered me, not Russ.

The IV pole wouldn't come until early the next week, so I wandered around the house looking for options. As I entered our bedroom, my face broke into a big smile. *Of course! My steam cleaner!*

I hated to iron, so I bought this neat little steam cleaner to keep in my closet. It had a metal hook that could support the IV bag. An extended pole adjusted up and down. It was on wheels in case he had to go to the bathroom. It was perfect.

As I got the supplies ready, I laughed away my nerves. I was about to administer my first medical treatment—with a steam cleaner. I felt like I needed a commercial. "Stanley Steamer here, we'll steam your bugs away, or the next treatment is free!" or, "Come to Stanley Steamer for your next IV. Our treatments are hot!"

I could see future Russ telling the story and laughing. Future Russ.

Unfortunately, present Russ didn't think it was funny. As soon as I walked toward him with the steamer in tow, he panicked.

"What the hell is that? . . . No one told me about this . . . Why should I do this? . . . I'm going to die anyway . . . Do you even know what the hell you're doing?"

Honestly, no. Half the time, I have no idea what the hell I'm doing.

For over an hour, he argued, and I explained, again and again and again. Ryan came upstairs looking for breakfast. I sent him back downstairs and fed him and Hailey in the basement to keep them away. I didn't want them to see this. Heck, I didn't want to see this.

Russ kept arguing and arguing, and his anger fueled my doubt. I tried to redirect him, but he wouldn't stop. I tried to walk away, but he followed me. I begged for space, but he wouldn't leave. Eventually, I couldn't take it anymore, and I broke down on my closet floor and cried.

When he first saw me crumble, he walked away, frustrated that he couldn't continue the argument. Minutes later, he returned, but the look on his face changed. He was different. It was as if my tears had awakened a new part of his brain. The softness in his eyes returned. He no longer saw me as his persecutor but as the woman he loved.

"I'm so sorry," he said. "I didn't mean to make you upset. Sometimes, I don't know how to stop myself. I'll do anything you want. Please stop crying."

Before, when I cried, I felt a dramatic release, almost like throwing up when you feel sick to your stomach. The emotions swelled inside me until my body couldn't contain them anymore. But once I cried it out, I felt relieved. Better. But this cry was different. This time I didn't feel better. In the end, there was no relief. Just more to do, more to endure.

We held each other, and I gathered myself. Russ said he was ready, and I grabbed the steamer and administered my first IV.

Despite our tumultuous morning, the rest of the day was quite nice. Russ spent the early afternoon power washing the driveway. He cleaned it two weeks ago, but it kept him busy, so I went with it. Later in the day, we hung out in the backyard with the kids and the dogs. Junior grew bigger and more coordinated every day, and his antics made the kids squeal with excitement. We played frisbee and enjoyed the sunshine. It was almost like being a normal family.

One thing I'd learned, however, was that normal didn't last long. The next day, as Russ got out of the shower, I noticed a large bruise on the back of his arm. I freaked.

Did the IV do this? I'm not a nurse. Did I do something wrong? What do I do now?

I took a deep breath. *Okay. Calm down. Look at it again. It looks like it's healing. It's yellow around the edges. It's not raised or hot to the touch.*

It seems like it's been there a few days, and I didn't notice because it's on the back of his arm and not near the PICC line.

I texted our nurse, Ashley, a photo along with the words "FLIPPING OUT." She called right away and calmed my fears.

"Don't worry, love," she said. "You didn't do it. You're doing fine. It looks like blood pooling from the procedure, but wow, I've never seen bruising like that. What did the doctor do to him?"

Russ had told me the doctor was rough, but I brushed it off. I never knew when to listen and when to ignore. But for now, I was relieved he was okay.

I hung up the phone and cataloged all the things I needed to do before the kids got home from school, one of which was another IV. I wasn't a particularly religious person, but one phrase kept repeating in my head. *Lord, please help me.*

12

War on the Woods

May 2018

Russ and I first moved to California in March of 2004. We drove Route 80 across the country, hauling a trailer full of the items we needed to survive a few months until Russ's house in New Hampshire sold. As we traveled through Reno and Tahoe, the green mesmerized me. Rolling hills of lush grass filled the truck windows, and I smiled with girlish excitement, knowing that this was our home for as long as we chose.

Unfortunately, I soon learned that the green would fade like a well-planned April Fool's joke. Within a week of being settled, the lush grass turned a dismal brown. Russ laughed at my naivety.

"You know they call California the Golden State for a reason," he joked.

"Golden? This isn't golden. It's just brown. They should call it the brown state," I retorted.

"That would be crappy marketing." He paused. "Get it, crappy?"

I rolled my eyes. "You know, sometimes your puns are worse than my dad's. Not your best work," I teased.

Over the next two years, I coveted the blessed two weeks in the spring and fall when the green returned. It was like a handshake between the different plant phyla. The trees budded with shades of green in the spring, but their splendor seemed to be at the grass's expense, which transformed into a dull and pervasive brown. Later, in the fall, the grass returned to its verdant self, but the trees lost their leaves one by one. There was only enough green on the palette for a brief overlap. The lush paradise that welcomed me to California existed less than ten percent of the year.

As much as I lamented my golden landscape, I didn't realize how much the green fueled my soul until we went to North Carolina. The dense forests and fescue lawns provided green for more than half the year. It brought comfort and immediately signaled that this was home.

Our neighborhood was a vast, single estate that had been divided into sixty multi-acre lots. Dense forests of maples, oaks, cedars, and sweetgums covered the landscape in green. Portions of the forest were harvested by the previous landowners, leaving the associated lots full of young loblolly pines. When I lived in New England, I loved pines. They provided green all year long and brought texture and interest to the barren landscape. But in North Carolina, the loblollies were straggly and often bare except for the top third. They were shallow-rooted and prone to falling over in even a mild hurricane. In our neighborhood, they served as a reminder of the beautiful hardwoods that once stood in their place. I developed a guttural disdain for pines, and their absence became a critical selection criterion as we searched for houses and lots.

The lot we selected had been untouched by humanity, and the old hardwoods formed a green backdrop over seventy-five feet tall. A downward slope on the back half of the property made it great for a basement and provided a lovely vantage point to overlook the dense forest. We fell in love with it, and other options only brought us back to this spot in the woods where our house seemed to belong.

The covered back porch was my favorite room in the house. It wasn't actually a room since the sides were open, but I guess that's why I loved it so much. The front of the house faced south, so even in the heat of summer, the porch was cool. With the basement floor below, we sat perched high among the branches. We watched as the birds, deer, and even wild turkeys shared our little plot of Earth.

But now, as I looked out over the beautiful sea of green, it no longer brought comfort. Fear overcame me. I knew what lurked in the woods. Every young tree, every bush, and every low-hanging branch wasn't a welcome swatch of green; it was a home for ticks. I pulled dozens of ticks off Russ after he worked in the yard. North Carolina wasn't supposed to be a hotspot for Lyme, but I knew that wasn't true. My neighbors down the street—their son had Lyme. The Driscoll's dog—he had Lyme. It was here. Suddenly, the family of deer and the rolling woods were no longer my friends.

It was May, and prime tick season was only beginning. My anxiety swelled every time we went outside. I covered the kids in bug spray whenever they went out to play. The smell of lemon and eucalyptus burned our nose hairs, and heaven forbid if we opened our mouths during the application process. Even inside, I didn't feel safe. A landscaped fence confined the dogs, but I still found ticks on their bellies and paws. I searched and sprayed them, but suddenly, a sweet dog asleep on my lap elevated my heart rate.

Then it happened. One Saturday morning, Hailey trounced down for breakfast after sleeping late. She was in a phase where she liked to sleep shirtless, so she whirled around the living room and kitchen like a half-dressed ballerina. She gave her morning hug to Junior and then sat at the kitchen table to feast on some paleo pancakes.

As she finished eating, she squealed. "Mom! There's a bug on me! Get it off, get it off!"

Her pitch was too grating for my one-coffee morning, but I grabbed a napkin and sprang into action. Sure enough, there was a bug crawling across her torso, and sure enough, it was a deer tick. It hadn't attached, but it was there, and if she hadn't been shirtless, we wouldn't have noticed.

I grabbed a Ziplock bag and cataloged the tick in my growing collection. I felt like a crazed entomologist who despised the subject of her study. Hailey calmed down, but my distress grew.

How can I live where I don't feel safe? Hailey hadn't been out in the woods. She came straight from her bed. The tick probably got on her when she hugged Junior, which of course, meant they could be *anywhere* in the house. The dogs were all over the couches, the blankets, our beds, everywhere. I couldn't live in constant fear twenty-four hours a day.

As Hailey settled into her morning cartoons, I drank my second cup of coffee on the deck overlooking the cursed woods. *Damn ticks. You've stolen my husband, and now, you're stealing my freaking house. Well, fuck you. I'm not letting you have them. I'm healing my husband, and I'm taking my house back.*

And that was the moment I officially declared my war on the woods.

Within two days, my new landscaper came over and reviewed the plan. I wanted all green within fifteen feet of the ground gone: young plants, weeds, branches, all of it. We wouldn't touch the big trees other than trimming the low branches, but everything else must go. I started with a small area right outside the fence, but it looked so clean and wonderful that I quickly expanded to the side yard and deeper into the woods. By the time I was done, nearly two acres of the lot were open at the bottom. Aesthetically, it looked better. Instead of an untamed melee of overgrown weeds, it was a beautiful forest. The stream running through the side of the property was now uncovered and visible from the yard. A bit of peace started to return, but I still wasn't done.

Next, I covered the property with Tick Control Tubes. Most people only think of ticks on deer, but they attach to all animals. Young ticks, called nymphs, prefer to feed on mice. In endemic areas, a single mouse could have *sixty* parasitic little nymphs on board—what a disgusting thought. The tubes I bought were developed based on research at Harvard. Each tube contained cotton soaked in permethrin, a synthetic chemical that acts like natural extracts from the chrysanthemum flower and, most importantly, kills ticks. Mice collect the cotton and use it as bedding in their burrows. These permethrin-covered mice now eliminate young nymphs attempting to feed on them. I imagined each rodent as a highly lethal ninja assassin, carefully eradicating hundreds of young *Borrelia* factories.

Finally, I contracted a service to spray the yard with permethrin as a mosquito and tick repellent. I knew this spray could harm other insects like bees and fireflies, but this was war. I wanted every last tick off my property.

Almost immediately, I stopped seeing ticks on the dogs. I was still vigilant, but my anxiety faded, at least around the house. Of course, I wouldn't let the kids leave the garage without their plume of protection, and the dogs weren't allowed to walk in the tall grass that often adorned the edge of vacant lots. The battle was still on, but I claimed my high ground.

* * *

As it turned out, Scott waged another war on the woods with a very different strategy. I told him about Hailey's crawling critter the following Monday on my way to work.

"I know what you mean," he said. "We won't even sit on the grass at baseball games anymore. We're the crazy people sitting back on the sidewalk or parking lot because the grass freaks us out. It makes Jodi hyperventilate sometimes."

I was glad to hear I wasn't the only one losing my mind. Everyone else seemed to live in a carefree bubble, and I often felt like the only one who saw the world for what it was, a biological bloodbath.

He went on. "It's so bad that we're considering moving. Virginia is rampant with Lyme, and we don't feel safe here anymore."

I was stunned. "Seriously? Where would you go?"

"We're looking at Scottsdale. I've got friends out there, and I can open a new office. Arizona still has ticks, but there aren't many in the desert. It's too hot, and they dehydrate too fast. I want my family to sit outside and relax for a change."

"But what about the business?" Scott built a successful practice in Virginia focused on aesthetics and wellness. I couldn't imagine him starting over.

"I'll keep my practice in Virginia and travel back and forth. It'll be hectic, but once everything is up and running, it should be easier. And I'll make sure the staff is self-sufficient and doesn't need a lot of hand-holding."

"Wow. That's huge. I can't believe it," I said.

"Well, I always wanted to retire to Scottsdale anyway. Moving now will be even better since I'll have the business and can work as long as I want. Plus, we won't be surrounded by ticks all the time."

He paused. "You know, Nick, I'll only say this once because it's your decision, but if you want to be free of Lyme, you've got to get out of that house. Otherwise, it will always be with you."

I knew he was right. I couldn't step outside without worrying. And if the ticks weren't enough, we also had mosquitoes and their long list of infectious diseases. Living by the lake surrounded by forest came with a colossal downside. Somehow, I no longer felt like the top of the food chain.

"You may be right," I said. "But like I always say to Russ, we don't make big decisions on bad days. I'm barely keeping afloat now. Add a move, and you'll have more than your family to take care of."

He laughed. "Well, I'll keep you posted. I have to run to my first appointment, but we'll catch up later. Love you."

"Love you too."

As I hung up the phone, I didn't know what to think. I'd never considered moving. I used to joke with Russ that I'd be buried somewhere in the backyard. It was my forever home. Or was it?

I stopped myself. *We don't make big decisions on bad days. We don't make big decisions on bad days.*

13

Sorting Symptoms

May - July 2018

I'd worn a lot of different hats in my career. Engineering, business development, marketing. I'd done them all multiple times in various types of companies. Jack of all trades but master of none. On some levels, that label rang true. I wasn't an expert in any one area. My true passion emerged when I reached across multiple disciplines and made them work better together.

I guess that's why I kept landing in program management. Since I played various roles, seeing different perspectives came naturally. People who thought differently weren't a problem; they were an asset. The right answer could often be found within the team, waiting for the courage to be communicated. After all, poor communication topped the reasons why teams and projects failed. I'd seen it countless times in projects I was brought in to fix.

Being a caregiver was new to me, but working with people and problems wasn't. I tried to see parallels between my work with Russ and my work in the office. The doctor was now my program manager in the most important project I'd ever undertaken. How could I make his job easier? What did I appreciate most about the people and teams that worked for me?

The first thing that came to mind was data: garbage in equals garbage out. If the inputs and methods were bad, there was no way to make a good decision. People gravitated toward the things they believed in and missed the things that didn't fit their framework. Without data, there was only bias.

The ups and downs of treatment were insane. To say things varied from day to day was an understatement. Most days, they varied by the hour. One minute Russ was delighted to watch Ryan play baseball, and the next, he flew off the handle and threatened to drive to Atlanta. There was no way to be objective in the middle of it. I needed to record everything. I needed logs.

At first, I started with a daily log on the computer, but I soon realized I needed a more real-time solution. If there was a subtle change or comment, I wanted to write it down immediately before the madness of life made me forget to document it. So, I downloaded a symptom tracker on my phone and logged everything I could think of: the food he ate, the pills he took, the symptoms he experienced, and his overall behavior and mood. A good project manager keeps track of everything, at least until they know the metrics that matter.

Pretty soon, pages and pages of information spit out of my printer. It was overwhelming. In the engineering world, those who brought pages and pages of data with no analysis got sent back to their cubes. For the data to be useful, I needed to search for trends.

We were about to meet with Dr. Parker, so I spent an afternoon reviewing my logs a few days before our appointment. I picked a day when Russ was busy in the yard, so I could sit and think objectively. When did his symptoms flare or subside? Was there a common thread behind his triggers? Did some medicines impact him more than others? I searched each post and collection of posts for clues. I uncovered insights I never noticed in the day-to-day.

Once I analyzed the data, I needed to distill the findings into a digestible format. The longer appointment times at Dr. Parker's office were a nice change from the fast-food model of traditional medicine. But still, how could I maximize our time? Six weeks of life was a lot to communicate, and my logs and research left nothing but questions. I sat down and wrote a four-page email with a bulleted list of comments. Each high-level bullet contained a summary phrase. Then, the bullets underneath housed supporting observations and follow-up questions. It was how I wanted someone to communicate to me, so why wouldn't I do that for the doctor who held the keys to Russ's health?

When we went to our appointment, I felt prepared despite the chaos. The honeymoon period with Dr. Parker was over, and Russ saw the visit as another forced appointment. The cuss words flowed, and two breathing breaks kept me from spiraling into a nervous breakdown.

When Dr. Parker entered the exam room, he held my email. He smiled as he sat down.

"First, I want to say thank you for your email. I can't tell you how helpful this is to get up to speed on how you've been doing. I read it yesterday. Maybe we can go through each high-level bullet one by one?"

"That sounds great," I replied, relieved. My experience with Dr. Shit Happens was still fresh. He'd ignored my email, so I'd wondered how Dr. Parker would react to my pages of notes. *He read it and appreciated it. Maybe we finally have a partner in this process.*

"Okay, let's see . . . the first one. The two weeks off antibiotics was a very rough period. It seems like the aches and pains returned, you experienced fatigue, shortness of breath . . ."

As he talked, Russ squirmed in his seat. He gripped the chair so hard that his knuckles turned white. Russ's distress was contagious, but Dr. Parker was immersed and missed our cues. He went on.

"There was also a lot of confusion, constantly losing things. You had trouble with even basic tasks like the dishes . . ."

Russ couldn't take it anymore.

"This is ridiculous!" he shouted. "Confused? I may be a lot of things, but I am *not* confused. And if you don't like the way I do the damn dishes, then you do them!"

The subtle cues became a massive cue stick that whacked Dr. P. on the head. I shot him the same ice queen laser stare I often used to warn Ryan that Dad was in a mood.

"How about we focus on your observations and what we can do to make things better rather than reviewing every note?" I suggested. My laser stare let him know it wasn't optional.

"Of course." He nodded and then reviewed silently. "I see you had a lot of dizziness. Are you drinking enough water?"

I looked at Russ to draw him back into the conversation.

"Probably not, right? What do you think, Russ?" I asked.

"I don't know. I drink a couple of glasses a day," he replied. He was still tense, but the pink returned to his fingers.

"You need to be sure you're drinking a lot more water than usual to help flush your system. Perhaps we can add an IV lactated ringer a few times a week? It's basically water with electrolytes to keep you hydrated. Sound good?"

Russ nodded.

We kept going, and Dr. Parker attempted to include him in the conversation in a positive way. By the end of the appointment, Russ's demeanor changed, and he joked around and smiled.

As we walked out of the office, I saw the value in my summary. I prided myself in seeing different perspectives, but I forgot the one that mattered most: Russ. I wanted to give the doctor the information, but I never realized how demoralizing it was for Russ to sit there and hear me talk about all his issues. I described the loss of his decision-making skills, short-term memory, and word-finding. With every spoken word, he felt more broken. The written summary helped the doctor and me, but most importantly, it helped Russ maintain a bit of dignity.

From then on, it became a way of life: log, analyze, and summarize—a nice tool to organize the confusion of our lives.

During this process, I noticed some themes. One central theme was that *Bartonella* was as ugly as Lyme, at least in Russ's case.

We were stable on the second round of antibiotics. Russ's pains were gone, his mood was pretty even, and his energy was high. Then on week five of the six-week protocol, we ran out of one of the antibiotics: Rifabutin. I didn't think much of it since our appointment with Dr. Parker was only a few days away, and I knew he'd renew the script. Russ was on eight different antibiotics. Missing one of them for a few days couldn't hurt anything, right? If only that were true.

Russ missed his Monday and Wednesday doses, and by Thursday morning, he was a mess. The pain in his arm returned, he complained of back pain, he felt severe fatigue, and his mood fluctuations came back in full force. New symptoms also emerged. He complained of urinary pain and lack of control, and red, itchy sores covered his lower legs. It was worse than when he went off all antibiotics, but the only thing we'd changed was one little pill.

I emailed Dr. Parker, and he called in a new prescription. When he'd first prescribed it, I balked at the price: $295 for thirty pills. After seeing Russ suffer, I'd pay almost anything to get another bottle. Russ took a dose on Thursday evening, and by Friday, everything stabilized. Well, Russ stabilized; I still felt like fresh tornado debris.

When we met with Dr. Parker for our scheduled appointment, he explained that the Rifabutin treated the *Bartonella*. Russ's response clearly showed that *Bartonella*, or Bart for short, was a significant contributor in his case. As I researched, it made sense. Bart was associated with mood instability, rage, depression, fatigue, and muscle pain. It all fit. I'd blamed his depression and anger on so many things over the years. I wondered how much of it was Bart rearing its ugly head.

Instead of taking a break from antibiotics after week six as planned, Dr. Parker suggested we stay on the meds for another two weeks. He also wanted to try an herbal therapy designed to target *Bartonella*. We went home with a tiny tincture vial. He warned that these tinctures were potent and started Russ on one drop mixed in an ounce of water.

I looked at the ingredients: Cat's Claw, Sarsaparilla, Pau d'Arco, Burdock, Blessed Thistle, Mullein Leaf, and Oregon Grape Root. It seemed ridiculous. Russ took buckets of pills twice a day, but *one drop* of this witch's brew would make a difference? I didn't see it. Again, I was wrong.

I waited until Russ recovered from the Rifabutin debacle, and then I gave him one drop in the morning and one in the evening. The next day he woke up complaining of lower back and knee pain. He was also agitated and depressed. His urinary control issues returned, as did the rash. I was flabbergasted, but I still wasn't convinced.

I stopped the drops for a few days and watched his symptoms subside. Then, like a mad scientist wondering what my next ingredient would bring about, I gave him a drop at night. He woke up upset and complained that his back ached. As evening came, he grew calmer, and his pain eased. It was unreal. One drop. It defied science—or at least the science that I knew.

Again, I reached out to Dr. Parker. He recommended backing off to 1/4 of a drop in the morning and evening. He also stepped up Russ's detox protocol. Skeptical, I complied, and I documented. Russ was still irritable, but it was more tolerable. We could manage. After about four days, the dose didn't impact Russ at all, at which point Dr. Parker recommended we up his dose by another 1/4 drop. He said we should keep increasing the dose until Russ could tolerate fifteen drops twice a day. I could gradually increase to whatever he could handle.

Jodi also suffered from Bart, so I reached out to ask about her experience. It was a timely question since she was also in the middle of a *Bartonella*-focused protocol. It was different from Russ's, but there were some parallels. Her text messages left me numb.

"Nick, Bart is a serious bitch. I've been through protocols for Lyme and *Babesia*, and I haven't experienced *anything* like this. Yesterday, I was so freaking paranoid. I don't even know why, but I felt paralyzed. I sat curled up in a ball in the corner of my bedroom for almost two hours. I was completely wigging out. The anxiety is insane!"

Then she sent a photo with a simple question. "Has Russ ever had something like this?"

The photo was of a red sore that looked irritated. The scratch marks next to it showed that it was itchy. I immediately knew that's what Russ had on his legs, but for some reason, at that moment, the rest of the picture hit me. Why hadn't I put it together before? Our Rifabutin flare wasn't the first time I'd seen that rash. I'd seen it many, many times.

Bugs seem to love certain types of people, and Russ was one of them. The two of us would go into the woods, and if I came out with one mosquito bite, he came out with twenty. Russ joked about his sweet blood and tried to take precautions. But every summer, he came in from yard work covered with bites. He scratched his legs like a flea-ridden dog.

"Damn chiggers," he said. He used bug spray religiously, but it never seemed to work. He even bought 100% DEET and sprayed it all over his legs, but the chigger bites got worse. I never understood it. The kids and I walked all over the grass with no bug spray and never got bites, but somehow, Russ was chigger bait.

Once I saw the picture, I looked at the same events through a different lens. The chigger bites looked like the *Bartonella* rash. What if they weren't chigger bites at all? What if all that DEET triggered his *Bartonella* to flare? Had it been right in front of me all along? What other symptoms did I miss?

I racked my brain. In 2008, before Ryan was born, we were building the house and living in a three-bedroom apartment. Russ was working for a company that made memory chips for cell phones. He called me at work around 10:00 a.m.

"Nikki, I'm in the stairwell at work. I need you to come get me. My heart is going crazy. I feel like I'm going to pass out."

"Are you serious? Holy shit. Can you get to the parking lot or no?"

"Yeah, I think I can. Meet me by the side door. And call the cardiologist."

I raced over to get him and drove immediately to his cardiologist's office. They checked him out and said he was okay. It was probably a panic attack, and they said we should let them know if it happened again. It didn't make sense because Russ had never had a panic attack before. But the doctor said he was fine, and we believed him. It never happened again, so we brushed it off as a weird experience.

A quick web search highlighted panic attacks as symptoms of Lyme, *Bartonella*, and other tick-borne illnesses. That was 2008. *Ten years ago.* If we'd only dug deeper then, I wondered where we'd be now.

14

Hope

May - July 2018

Scott and I started talking on the phone about once a week. We swapped notes on progress or the lack thereof; we vented frustrations and concerns; we shared new papers and resources. It was like group therapy and a scientific journal club all wrapped into a thirty-minute call. I'd never been close to my brother, so it was a much-needed bright side that our hardships brought us closer together.

Jodi was on antibiotic therapy for almost a year, and it wore on both of them.

"I don't know, Nick," he said. "It seems to get harder and harder. This Bart protocol is killing her. I'm not sure she's going to be able to stay on it much longer."

"So, what are you going to do?" I asked.

"Well, the last couple of months, I've been researching alternate therapies. Things that focus on building your immune system and letting it do the killing rather than antibiotics. One thing that looks promising is stem cell therapy."

I remembered studying stem cells while I was at Duke. Clinical use was typically limited to autologous transplants in a localized area, like a joint. That meant stem cells from the patient were harvested and amplified, then injected back into the patient to stimulate repair and growth. It was FDA approved and practiced across the county.

But more aggressive attempts using stem cells had some notable failures. A woman grew nasal tissue on her spine when researchers attempted to use olfactory stem cells to repair nerve damage. The headline "Nose Grown on Woman's Back" wasn't exactly comforting. I also had the disgusting images of teratomas from embryonic stem cell transplants stuck in my brain forever. Tumors made up of different tissue types flashed before my eyes: hair, muscle, teeth, bone. It was a buffet of nastiness captured in gut-wrenching dissection photos. Stem cell therapy could mean many things, and I had no idea what flavor captured Scott's interest.

"Really?" I asked. "What kind of stem cell therapy?"

"I'm looking at stem cells from Wharton's jelly. You know, the gelatinous substance found in umbilical cords. Most clinical stem cell work is done with autologous transplants, mainly because transplants from other donors get rejected, like in organ transplants. Well, as it turns out, the stem cells in Wharton's jelly don't express the molecules that lead to rejection. It's part of the reason that the mom's immune system doesn't reject the baby, and they can exchange so much material via the umbilical cord. Their immune privilege allows transplants from other donors."

"Huh, that's interesting," I said, taking it all in. "What kind of stem cells are they?"

"They're Mesenchymal Stem Cells, or MSCs."

"Like in bone marrow?" I asked.

"Yes, exactly," he answered. "But they're easier to collect and seem to be more potent than bone marrow-derived cells. Also, Wharton's jelly has a ton of growth factors and cytokines that stimulate the immune system. I've been talking to a doctor in California who's performed IVs on hundreds of people, including Lyme patients. She sees great results."

"Results like what?"

"Less fatigue, reduced pain, better immune system function. It's helping people get better faster." He paused. "I'm thinking we're going to give it a try on Jodi."

I had pulled into the parking lot at work and started to get my things out of the car, but his comment stopped me dead in my tracks.

"Damn. You're that sure?"

"I think so. I've been reading about it for a while now, and my contact is already using it clinically. The only real downside is the risk of infection, but if you use a reputable donor lab, the risk of infection is low. Jodi has been a mess lately, and we need to try something different."

"Wow. Well, keep me posted. It sounds fascinating. And send me some papers I can read. You know me."

He laughed. "Will do. I've got to run, but we'll catch up later."

A couple of weeks later, Jodi had the stem cell treatment. The first several days were rough, but she hit an inflection point on day ten and felt better than she had in years. Usually, getting out of bed and going to the bathroom drained her, but after the treatment, she felt good enough to take the dogs for a walk. Her anxiety was gone, and she finally could get a good night's sleep. She texted me her daily progress, and I was fascinated. I stepped up my research and prepared for my next call with Scott.

"Okay, so I think my biggest question is, do the stem cells cross the blood-brain barrier?" I asked. Of all my questions, it was the most important. Russ's battleground was the brain.

"I asked about this as well," Scott replied, "and for neuro cases, they give an IV beforehand that temporarily destabilizes the blood-brain barrier. That way, the cells can penetrate. Of course, there's no real way to know how many make it, but the results are encouraging."

"So, she sees a cognitive benefit with her patients?"

"She does, but at this point, it is more anecdotal than scientific. There are Alzheimer's trials going on in Mexico right now. They won't publish the results for years, but they're looking at it. Plus, even if the stem cells don't cross the blood-brain barrier, the growth factors will. That won't last as long, but it can still be therapeutic."

"So, what do you think?" I knew what his answer would be, but I needed to hear it out loud.

"Honestly, I think you should do it. It's made a big impact on Jodi, and you're already behind the eight ball with Russ."

He was right. Even with all our progress on physical symptoms, his cognitive performance continued to decline. I tried to convince myself otherwise, but the logs didn't lie.

For the next several days, I agonized. I'd departed from mainstream medicine a while back, but this was even further on the fringe. At work, I spent all day coordinating study after study to prove that our devices were safe and effective. The FDA scrutinized every report and summary and decided what was allowed and considered "on label" use. This use of stem cells was clearly off label, something that—as a device manufacturer—was hammered into my head as being bad. But for doctors, it was at their discretion and risk. It was a big fat gray area.

Do I want to experiment on my husband? The thought repeated in my head. I once again watched Russ help with the dishes, a task that used to be exclusively his. He washed a plate, raised it above the counter, and stopped. He stared, studying it. The puzzled look on his face told me he couldn't remember whether he washed it and needed to put it in the dishwasher or if he took it out of the dishwasher and needed to put it in the cabinet.

Desperate times. Desperate measures.

Dr. Parker didn't perform the stem cell treatments, so Scott helped me get all the materials to do it at home through the PICC line. I waited until Russ was on week five of his antibiotic protocol. That way, I expected his symptoms and mood to be stable, and I also had enough time to monitor the effects before our two weeks off. I was ready—or as ready as I could be.

On the day of the treatment, I was nervous. I had the protocol, and I knew what to do, but I couldn't get rid of the incessant what ifs that rattled in my head. Russ knew we were trying something a bit crazy and was all for it.

"Why not?" he said. "I'm going to die anyway, so why not try it and see what happens? Medical research at its best!"

His cavalier attitude made me feel better and worse at the same time.

After the treatment, we waited. Two days later, Russ woke up, and his penis, which had been dangling for months, was wonderfully and beautifully erect. We had settled into a routine of being roommates or caregiver and patient, depending on the day. I figured it was his low testosterone, but I was afraid to put him on replacement therapy while his mood was unstable. The last thing I needed was a dementia patient with roid rage. But all of a sudden, he was on like a switch, and he couldn't keep his hands off me. We reconnected, again and again. It refueled every cell in my body.

Whatever stoked his sex drive didn't trigger any other notable improvements, at least initially. Most of the week following treatment, word-finding and conversations were more difficult than usual. He was also fatigued but in a weird way. Instead of sleeping, he sat on the couch as if in a trance. It was as if his soul left, and a zombie took over. As I began to wonder if the treatment did more harm than good, Russ hit an inflection point. Like with Jodi, it was on day ten.

It was Saturday morning, and Ryan and Hailey were playing a game of apple sauce soccer in the foyer. I spent hundreds of dollars on toys, yet their favorite game was soccer using a cap from one of their apple sauce pouches as a ball. Russ walked in from the garage, and I braced myself for the explosion. Hailey screeched in delight as she scored a goal, and tension shot through my shoulders. As I devised my plan to shuffle them to the basement, Russ walked to the foyer. I followed him, analyzing nine different damage control scenarios in my brain.

Instead, as he got there, his stare softened. He smiled. Before I knew it, he jumped in, got a pass from Hailey, and kicked it to the front door, also known as the goal. He picked her up and twirled her around as she screamed, "More! More!"

Ryan piled on and pleaded for a piggyback ride. Again, I prepared for the worst. Surely the two kids clamoring for his attention would lead to disaster. But instead, he grabbed Ryan, threw him on his back, and chased Hailey around the house like a double-headed monster.

Later at dinner, the kids chatted away about their play date with our neighbors, the Driscolls. As I tried to pay attention to the blow-by-blow narrative of the afternoon's events, I noticed Russ staring at me. The look in his eyes transported me back to our late-night business trip dinners years ago. He smiled and reached to grab my hand; his gaze fixated. Finally, Hailey, known for saying whatever was on her mind, noticed that she didn't have our focus.

"Are you guys even listening, or are you just going all googly-eyed on each other?"

Russ and I laughed and turned our attention back to their stories. She was so much like me: strong, stubborn, and brutally honest. Ryan was so much like Russ: charming, sweet, and adorably funny. We made so much good. If only we could see our way to the other side of this mess.

The next few weeks, I saw snippets of what my life could be and should have been. In between all the pills and anger and tears, I'd almost forgotten.

Russ was calmer and happier. He laughed more, played more, and was more affectionate. Instead of coming up to my office and snapping about something broken or "fucked" up, he came to bring me a cup of coffee. He snuck behind me while I made dinner to hug me and tell me he loved me. The man I married was returning.

He also rediscovered the guitar. Russ started playing the guitar when he was twelve years old. His family barely got by financially, so Russ didn't have the plethora of activities that our kids enjoyed. Outside of school, he had a lot of time on his hands. His older brother, Ray, turned to drugs and made life miserable for Russ and Doug. Ray's pursuits led to all sorts of violence, the worst of which was a drive-by shooting at their house where a bullet missed nine-year-old Doug—who was asleep in his bed—by about twelve inches. Then, when Russ was a teenager, Ray pulled a gun on him during an argument. Russ escaped by jumping out of a second-story window. Needless to say, Russ didn't have a soft, comfy suburban life. In all the turmoil, Russ could have turned to disastrous pursuits. But he turned to the guitar instead.

A local music store captured Russ's interest, and he convinced his mom to buy him his first guitar. Most kids practiced for thirty minutes and called it a day. But Russ wasn't most kids. He practiced for *hours*, averaging six to seven hours a day. He told me this when we were dating, and I brushed it off as an exaggeration. No one could practice that much, especially a kid. I was a colossal overachiever, and I never came close to that kind of effort on anything. But sure enough, after we moved into our house, Russ came across his practice log in a big box of files as we unpacked. I flipped through the pages. Monday 7.5 hours, Tuesday 6 hours, Wednesday 8 hours, Thursday 5 hours, Friday 5.5 hours. It went on and on. He logged his practice time every day for *years* in a stack of loose-leaf lined paper. I pictured a little version of him jammed in his bedroom closet with only music to shield out the chaos.

It was the guitar that drew Russ to his career in electronics. Guitar gear was expensive, and Russ couldn't afford to buy a new amplifier at the store. He found a build-it-yourself kit and invested in that instead. The instructions were well beyond his prepubescent education, so Russ checked out library books on circuits to figure it out. While other kids rode bikes or played baseball, Russ sorted and connected transformers, capacitors, and vacuum tubes until his prized amplifier was complete.

Then, as his skills grew, he became fascinated with Johnny Winter. One of the guys at the music store bet that Russ couldn't learn one of Johnny's riffs by the end of the month. The guy thought it was a sure bet since he knew that Johnny's lightning-fast fingers had help from his love of amphetamines.

Of course, that didn't deter Russ. He searched his electronics books and built an adjustable voltage regulator to slow his tape deck's motor speed. He practiced at quarter-speed, then half-speed, then three-quarter speed. Eventually, he nailed the riff and won the bet. When he became the first in his family to go to college, his path was clear—electrical engineer by day and jazz musician by night.

When we designed the house, we built a guitar room right off the main living area, so Russ could play whenever the mood struck. On the back wall, three alcoves housed guitars. On the left was a 1968 SG Gibson Guitar that he bought used when he was seventeen years old. To purchase it, he saved for over two years and then logged tens of thousands of hours on it, practicing and playing with his first band. In the middle was a Sunburst Les Paul. He bought that one in his thirties while rising through the ranks in a top-tier electronics company. His boss at the time didn't appreciate that Russ often corrected him during meetings. When bonuses came out, Russ got the bare minimum, a fraction of his previous earnings. Russ spent the entire check on a guitar in a futile act of spite. It became his favorite, and he joked that it was the only good thing that boss ever gave him. Finally, on the right was a Fender Stratocaster that he bought during a blues phase in his forties. The room was once alive with late-night concerts and personalized jam sessions, but recently, the room remained dark.

As Russ started to feel better, he gravitated back to the guitar. One day, the lead line to "Black Magic Woman" drew me out of my office. He was playing the notes from memory on his Fender. One by one, he plucked the strings in a way that seemed familiar yet foreign. Typically, he played with a CD to jam along with the band, but the player was off.

"Do you want me to put on the CD?" I asked as I entered the music room.

"Yeah, do you think you can find it?"

"Definitely. It should be over here in this stack of your old jamming CDs." I searched and found it in the middle of the pile. "Here it is."

I slid the Santana disc into the player and advanced to the right track. His eyes closed, and the music overtook him. His fingers, after countless hours of practice, knew exactly what to do. At first, he played Carlos's part, mirroring him riff for riff. But eventually, Russ interjected more notes around the melody. His speed and artistry outpaced the band and reflected not only the hours he'd put in but also the way that music ignited him.

"I hear more notes than most people," he'd say with a somewhat cocky smile.

Once again, music filled our house. Santana, Stevie Ray Vaughn, Pat Metheny, and Atlanta Rhythm Section replaced the incessant noises of weed whackers, power washers, and blowers. The kids and I sat in the music room, watching Russ play. The speed of Russ's fingers captivated Ryan, but I focused on the passion and emotion that poured through his body. This was a pleasure I'd almost forgotten.

I used to envision Russ teaching the kids all that he knew. How to play the guitar, how to fix things around the house, how to change the oil in his car, how to test and debug circuits. Whatever he did, the kids would be in tow. But it wasn't always clear whether Russ wanted to have more children. Early in our relationship, we came to a turning point. I was twenty-seven and knew that kids were a must for me. I couldn't imagine a life without chubby cheeks and skinned knees. Giving that up would be giving up a part of me. As much as I loved Russ, I would walk away if what he wanted was different.

Russ was forty-seven and had a daughter in her twenties. The possibility of having more kids was a page long turned over. When I thrust the decision upon him, it unearthed a deep turmoil. His model of family was broken at a young age. His father was always absent, even when he was home. Ray tortured Russ and Doug in every waking moment, and their father did nothing to intervene. Russ was determined to get away from his family, and his indignation sparked his ambition and independence. He made his way out, but the emotions festered.

At twenty-three, Russ married the singer in his band. The physical attraction was strong, but it soon became apparent how different they were. They fought all the time, leaving their marriage in ashes and his relationship with his daughter broken and raw. Every time he connected with his daughter, it only seemed to encourage their differences, much like his ex. Regret over this relationship clouded the conversations about our future. So much failure. Why do it again?

But years of therapy after the divorce taught him how to deal with his emotions. He was more mature, more in control. We talked for hours about what he wanted for the rest of his life. Kids had to be something *he* wanted, not something he did for me. Night after night, he ruminated.

Then one afternoon, while walking through the North End in Boston, he grabbed both of my hands and said, "Let's do it."

Three months later, we moved to California.

Once we settled into our life in North Carolina, we prepared for parenthood. Russ bragged to all his friends about becoming Mr. Mom. He saw our family as a second chance—a chance to get it right. And in the early days, it often felt right. Russ slept on the floor in Ryan's room, allowing me to sleep while he calmed the cranky toddler. He patiently taught Ryan to ride his bike, a task that I failed to do on multiple occasions. Father-son outings at the shooting range brought lessons on ballistics and gun safety and secret trips to the store for treats Mom didn't allow. And they developed a list of their favorite shows—*Bugs Bunny, The Three Stooges, Gilligan's Island*—which they watched while snuggling and sharing popcorn. But when Russ's illness set in, the moments faded. Hindsight revealed that by the time Hailey was born, his disease was entrenched.

But now, the father we both envisioned seemed to be back. Russ rekindled his relationship with Ryan, and the two of them became inseparable. I watched as my weekends morphed into something more peaceful. One Saturday morning, they decided to wash my car. It started as a lesson, not unlike Mr. Miyagi with Daniel-san. But when it became time to rinse, that lesson turned into a massive water fight. Ryan ran around the car to provide cover from the onslaught. He tried to be stealthy, but Russ's antics made him laugh and revealed his position. The eight-year-old and the sixty-one-year-old ended up soaked.

Later that afternoon, they biked along the trail that Russ made through the backyard. Russ taught Ryan to jump roots and dodge rocks, something Ryan wasn't sure of at first. After a few laps, Ryan's confidence grew, and before long, the two of them zipped around the yard. Finally, just before dinner, they sat on the deck and spotted birds with Russ's binoculars. As dusk settled, they hunted for the sounds of whippoorwills and the flashes of fireflies. Ryan's smile was a younger version of the smile beaming back at him.

And Ryan had been improving too. He finished his Brain Balance program, and for the past few months, he was a different kid. His constant need to fidget and dominate the conversation subsided, and a calm, sweet little boy emerged. If I was upset or overwhelmed, he came over, hugged me, and asked how he could help. Instead of fighting over vegetables, he gobbled them up and asked for seconds. He earned merits at school for being prepared, helpful, and paying attention. His grades improved, and he had his sights set on moving up a level in math. I was amazed. Maybe my two Bell boys finally got the help they needed.

While Ryan was off with Dad, I enjoyed beautiful moments with Hailey. One afternoon she asked if we could read together. We went up to her room, and she thrust *The Cat in the Hat* in my lap. Ryan finally gifted his coveted books to her, and she immersed herself in a Dr. Seuss phase.

After I finished the book, she asked, "Can I read you one now?"

I was a bit surprised since she still struggled with reading, but I checked myself and encouraged her. "Of course! Why don't you go pick the book."

She walked over to her bookshelf and studied each title. I expected her to grab one of the simple readers we practiced with, but instead, she came back with *Green Eggs and Ham.*

"This one!" she exclaimed with a huge grin on her face.

"Oooh . . . my favorite. But it's a long one. Are you sure you're up for it?"

"Yup," she said.

She snuggled up next to me and put her finger under the first word as they taught her in school. Word by word, she tracked with her finger and sounded them out. I was astonished as she read the first page, then the next, then the next. Before I knew it, she read the entire book. Of course, some words took help, but not as many as I thought. And her persistence was epic. When Ryan first started to read, he did great initially but then conked out and asked me to finish. Hailey read page by page without any signs of frustration or fatigue—only tenacity. As she closed the book, a smile connected her pudgy cheeks.

"Hailey Grace Bell, that was wonderful! You've been hiding your reading talents from me. What other skills are you hiding?"

"Well, let's see," she thought. "I can count to 109!"

"You can? Well, you know what? If you can count to 109, then you can also count to 110."

Later that night, Ryan and I decided to catch up on *Battlebots,* a TV show where 250-pound robots faced off in combat. The main event was Lock-Jaw versus Bronco, and we debated whether the vertical spinner or the pneumatic flipper would emerge victorious. We set up Hailey in the basement with her favorite cartoon, and the three of us got ready for Robot Fighting Time. Russ fell asleep about thirty minutes in, but Ryan and I were entranced. During the final battle, Bronco nearly flipped Lock-Jaw out of the arena, and Ryan hollered in excitement. His enthusiasm woke up Russ, and I was on edge after years of experience. But rather than scream and storm off, Russ got up, patted Ryan on the head, and went to bed.

When everyone was asleep, I sat in the living room and felt the warmth roll over me. Russ was finally responding well to treatment. He'd been through two rounds of antibiotics, and whether it was that or the stem cell treatment, I couldn't be sure, but it was clear we were on the right path. Even this last time off antibiotics wasn't bad. He got a little cranky a couple of times, but I gave him a lactated ringer, and he pulled out of it. His cognitive skills still weren't great, but once again, I saw the man I fell in love with staring back at me.

Plus, Ryan's success with Brain Balance spawned my new fascination with neuroplasticity. The books I read told tale after tale of the brain remapping itself after damage. Doctors were having success regenerating neurons using supplements to stimulate neurotrophins such as Brain-Derived Neurotrophic Factor, or BDNF. And who knew what we could do with stem cells? We finally had options. Russ might not be the engineer he was, but we could rebuild where we could. He could contribute around the house, help with the kids, and be a husband. I relaxed and allowed myself to hope.

15

Uncovering Illness

Lyme Crazy. I'd heard the term many times since entering the Lyme world, and it seemed to have a double meaning. First, chronic Lyme often has a psychological impact. Inflammation in the body and brain leads to imbalances in neurotransmitter and hormone levels. Patients become moody, belligerent, depressed, suicidal. Whatever the presentation, it isn't "normal." Maybe their behavior destroys their relationship and leads to divorce. Perhaps they can't meet the demands at work, and they lose their job. They used to be fine, but now, they're acting weird or crazy.

But there's also a powerful second meaning. Patients feel sick all the time, but doctors can't figure out why. Time after time, they walk into a doctor's office feeling terrible, only to be told they aren't sick at all. Perhaps it's in their head, and they need to seek psychiatric care. They see doctor after doctor, but no answers emerge. Meanwhile, their fatigue worsens and brings more pain, more isolation. Rejection after rejection makes patients *feel* crazy—gaslighted by a healthcare system that's supposed to help. No one listens. No one understands.

I didn't advertise Russ's illness. We were private people, and I wasn't ready for the barrage of interest and advice that came with widespread sharing. Nor was I hiding anything. Friends and coworkers often asked about our family and how we were doing. Most people asked to make conversation but didn't care about the answer. The last thing they wanted was the blow-by-blow of our painful reality. But some people inquired with sincere interest and asked a second or maybe a third question. With them, I shared our struggle.

I was surprised to discover that Lyme afflicted several people in our relatively small circle. Friends and coworkers had silently endured their struggle. When all was well in our household, I had no idea. But now that Lyme ravaged my family, the stories emerged. Before I knew it, over a dozen people shared their stories. Each tale made the harsh reality of being "Lyme Crazy" more and more clear.

Adryin

Adryin was the designer who helped decorate our newly finished basement. I asked my contractor to recommend a designer to make the construction process turnkey, and he introduced me to Adryin. I liked her immediately. She was at our house quite a bit and figured out that something wasn't right with Russ. She asked some questions about him and seemed genuine, so I told her our story. As soon as I mentioned Lyme, her eyes lit up.

Her story started in January of 2007. Out of the blue, she felt nauseous and couldn't get out of bed. Her sinuses ached, her head throbbed, and she lacked energy. She had a three- and a five-year-old, and she didn't have the strength to drive her youngest to preschool. The symptoms didn't subside, so after two weeks of agony, she went to the doctor. At the time, she didn't have a primary care physician, so she saw the nurse practitioner at her gynecologist's office.

The nurse reviewed her symptoms and asked what seemed like an odd question.

"Is there any chance you were bitten by a tick?"

Adryin was shocked. She lived in North Carolina, not New England, and it was the middle of the winter. But when she thought about it, she realized that she did have a weird bite right above her hip. She had developed a bit of a rash, but it wasn't the classic bullseye rash. She figured it was a flea bite from a stowaway on her dog.

They decided Lyme wasn't the culprit and treated her for the flu instead. She got some rest, took antivirals, and felt better. Two weeks later, she relapsed. Adryin went back to see the nurse practitioner, and once again, the NP mentioned Lyme. The nurse had Lyme herself, and Adryin's symptoms fit the picture. She referred her to Dr. Parker, but Adyrin was still skeptical. When she got home, she decided to straighten up her messy house with whatever energy she could muster. As she changed the sheets in her bedroom, she saw it—a dead tick.

Dr. Parker ran a battery of blood work. Adryin tested negative for Lyme, but much of her other blood work was off. She was almost anemic, her inflammation markers were high, and her hormone levels were perimenopausal even though she was only thirty-five. Her symptoms continued to worsen. She couldn't think clearly, was clumsy, suffered bouts of anxiety, and experienced shortness of breath. A few months earlier, she'd felt great and was killing it at the gym. Now, she was in a never-ending nosedive.

Despite the negative test result, Dr. Parker diagnosed her with Lyme and put her on three months of oral and IV antibiotics. Her family, including her husband, thought she was insane. She was treating a disease she didn't have; all the antibiotics would kill her immune system; the doctor was a quack. She heard it all. Her husband and mother chastised her every time she went for treatment, but Adryin persisted. She knew something was wrong, and the diagnosis made sense. Plus, as soon as she went on antibiotics, she felt better. Her fatigue subsided, the anxiety went away, her head cleared. If she didn't have the disease, then why was the treatment working so well?

Adryin stayed with Dr. Parker for about eighteen months. After her antibiotics, they restored her overall health with diet changes, vitamin and mineral supplements, and probiotics. She is now healthy, vibrant, and beautiful inside and out.

But her journey took its toll. Her illness stressed her marriage to its breaking point, and she filed papers of separation in 2009. Her mother still refuses to believe she had Lyme and calls her crazy whenever the topic arises. She remembers feeling so helpless, so judged. She wondered if she was losing her mind because everyone told her she was. Fortunately, her first stop was a healthcare provider who understood.

She found a doctor who believed her and helped her. She stuck with it, even when her closest family belittled her.

And today, she's well.

Phil

Phil was a team-building consultant I worked with for over five years. He served as a coach for my team and me, and we spent countless hours at off-site meetings, honing communication techniques and learning to appreciate each team member's strengths and weaknesses. Despite all our time together, I had no idea that one of Phil's strengths was that he had survived Lyme.

A colleague who knew Phil on a personal level was the first to clue me in. He suggested I give Phil a call to learn from his experiences, and so I did. Phil grew up out west and had been bitten by ticks many times while growing up, but he remembered a specific tick bite from 1999. While helping a friend with some work on his farm on the Maryland shores, he pulled a tick off his left shoulder. Later, the spot turned red. Phil figured it was infected, and he put rubbing alcohol on it until it got better. He'd heard of Lyme disease, but he never thought he might get it.

Phil went about his hectic life, and all seemed fine, but eventually, weird symptoms materialized. He experienced heart palpitations and had a hard time sleeping. He traveled a lot for work at the time, so he brushed it off as jet lag or stress. He also experienced burning in his feet, like he was walking on pins and needles. Again, he rationalized the symptoms and moved on.

In 2002, his symptoms got so bad he could barely sit up. His abdomen was sore, his legs and arms ached, and he couldn't sleep. He was a former NFL athlete and stayed in great shape, but now, his hands hurt him so much he couldn't even open a car door. He struggled to walk and to go up and down stairs. Something was wrong, and he went to the doctor to figure it out.

From 2002 to 2005, he saw dozens of doctors. None of them provided answers, but Phil kept pushing. Each new doctor checked him out, and each said that he was healthy. Maybe his problem was psychological. Still seeking answers, in 2004, he went to the Mayo

Clinic for an intensive executive physical. Surely, the brain trust there could figure out why he felt terrible all the time. Over four days, they ran panels and panels of tests, but they couldn't determine what was wrong. It was clear he had a mysterious blood infection, but that was all they knew.

Phil felt increasingly distraught. He was ordinarily outgoing and social, but now, he was withdrawn and isolated. He spent all his time in bed, and despite the exhaustion, he couldn't sleep.

In 2005, he saw a dermatologist for a weird rash on his body. Phil described his litany of symptoms, and she listened and asked probing questions. She then asked if doctors had ever tested him for Lyme and told him her story. This doctor was thirty-four years old and was an avid marathon runner. Suddenly, she'd started having hip problems, and before long, her orthopedist recommended a hip replacement. It didn't make sense, so she kept digging and researching and figured out that the root of her problem was Lyme. She went through treatment and was back to running without the need for a new hip. Phil's symptoms sounded like a classic case, and she recommended he see a doctor in New York to get an assessment.

It took over two months to get the appointment, but when he went, everything changed. The doctor sent out for blood work. There were only two labs in the United States that he trusted for accurate Lyme results. It turned out that Phil was positive for Lyme and *six* other tick-borne coinfections. The doctor put him on an intense course of rotating oral antibiotics for fourteen months. Slowly, symptom after symptom peeled away, and Phil felt like himself again. He now has lingering sleep issues and some neuropathy in his feet, but other than that, he's been healthy since he completed treatment in 2006. A fabulous story of recovery if it hadn't taken seven years.

Dierdre

Dierdre was a colleague who Russ and I worked with when we were in New Hampshire. We both loved her blunt honesty and snarky sense of humor and had kept in touch over the years. I hadn't spoken to Dierdre in a while, but I noticed when she posted a Lyme awareness article on

Facebook. I reached out and was sad to discover that Lyme had severely impacted her life.

Dierdre started having symptoms as early as 2001, when Russ and I worked with her. She experienced regular, debilitating headaches, and sporadically, her eyes flickered like a shutter closing on a camera. The world stopped for seconds or even minutes. Multiple doctors diagnosed her with epilepsy and put her on anti-seizure medication, but the drugs made her feel awful—like a zombie. She weaned off the meds and dealt with the return of her symptoms, which were manageable at the time.

In 2012, she became plagued with joint pain and digestive issues. Doctors diagnosed her with celiac disease, an immune condition that leads to damage of the small intestine after exposure to gluten. The pain lessened when she cut all gluten out of her diet, but it never went away. Determined to figure out her problem, she visited doctor after doctor. The best they offered was a diagnosis of fibromyalgia. They pushed her shoulder with two fingers, and when she confirmed that it hurt, they responded, "Yep, you have fibromyalgia." Frustration set in when the medication prescribed yet again made her feel worse. Her pain and sporadic seizures continued to worsen. She lost weight and had bouts of anxiety.

For the next five years, Dierdre struggled with the ebb and flow of symptoms. She was never tested for Lyme or coinfections, even though she had weird rashes twice. The first rash was in 2014, when she noticed an odd pattern on her neck. There was a dot in the middle, surrounded by dots all around. She was living in Illinois at the time, and the doctor diagnosed a spider bite and prescribed an antibiotic that worsened her joint pain. Then, in 2016, she felt ill and noticed a rash all over her stomach. A doctor examined her and said it was nothing worrisome.

Finally, in 2017, her neurological symptoms became debilitating. She stuttered when she spoke, misspoke words, and had trouble concentrating. Her new doctor worried that she had multiple sclerosis and ordered an MRI. Around the same time, her thyroid levels were off and weren't tracking with her medications, so she asked her endocrinologist for help. The endocrinologist suggested testing for Lyme and ordered an ELISA immunoassay and a Western Blot. The ELISA came back negative, and the Western Blot showed only three of the five bands needed for a positive diagnosis per CDC guidelines. Despite the negative results, her endocrinologist persisted. She ordered the urine PCR test from a specialty lab. That test indicated she was positive for Lyme, *Babesia*, *Bartonella*, and *Ehrlichia*. Almost sixteen years after her initial symptoms, she finally got answers.

Over the next year, Dierdre underwent treatment. She took multiple cycles of oral antibiotics, one course of IV antibiotics, and herbal protocols targeted for tick-borne infections. The treatment was rough at times, and her career suffered. Working remotely, she was often able to hide her symptoms, but when her boss demanded she take a role with more travel involved, she knew she couldn't handle it. The deadlock led to her termination, a fate that was foreign to her hardworking and diligent spirit.

Through persistence, Dierdre gradually returned to health. The antibiotics helped, but she also credits an herbal *Ehrlichia* protocol as a significant turning point. Three years later, Dierdre has no symptoms and lives in a new beach home with her supportive husband. She has a new job, her daughter lives nearby, and she bikes almost every day. She feels blessed that she found a doctor to heal her, and she lives each day with an earned appreciation for her health.

Clara

Clara and William lived in North Carolina, not too far from us. William worked for Russ when he ran the application engineering force for a major semiconductor company. Their job was to fix customer problems wherever they were, and William was one of the top guys called in for the hairiest situations. Russ loved everything about him except his "crazy" wife. Often when Russ needed William for a job, he couldn't go because Clara was sick. That happened over and over again. Russ didn't understand the problem; he only knew that it prevented William from doing his job.

One customer issue was so critical that Russ gave William an ultimatum.

"Get on the plane if you want to keep your job."

Somehow, William found help at home and made the trip. Russ moved on in his career and lost touch with William. But when William heard Russ had Lyme, he reached out. The four of us met for lunch, and we found out that "Crazy Clara" was Lyme Crazy.

Clara's journey started back in California in 1985, when she was pregnant with their second daughter, Amelia. During induced labor, Clara's placenta abrupted, which led to massive hemorrhaging. To make matters worse, the umbilical cord was wrapped around Amelia's neck three times. Both Clara and Amelia nearly died, but the doctors pulled them through. Amelia was perfect, and Clara was prescribed antibiotics for a uterine infection but was otherwise okay.

About a week later, Clara noticed that her hands and feet felt tingly and numb. She called her gynecologist and asked if the antibiotics could be causing her symptoms. She was told that her symptoms were unrelated, and when her condition worsened, they referred her to a neurologist.

The neurologist examined her and diagnosed her with transverse myelitis—an inflammation of the spinal cord. He told her to go home and rest for two months, an impossible task for the mother of an infant and a three-year-old child. When the doctor insisted, they asked William's mother to fly in from Missouri to take care of the girls. Clara rested but continued to get worse. The numbness traveled up her legs to her knees. Her arms felt so numb she didn't feel safe holding the baby, and she couldn't eat. She thought she was dying.

She saw neurologist after neurologist, but none of them could figure out what was wrong. They diagnosed her with multiple sclerosis and arranged a series of tests, the results of which caused them to conclude it wasn't MS after all. They referred her to specialist after specialist. Each one ran a new series of tests. Each one came back negative. Whatever it was, it wasn't something they could treat. Maybe try another specialty?

Doctors labeled her with symptomatic diagnoses like chronic fatigue syndrome and fibromyalgia. Some doctors found these diagnoses sufficient, while others laughed at the absurdity of chronic fatigue as an answer. Finally, they referred her to a psychiatrist because the problem had to be in her head. The psychiatrist did an extensive examination and concluded that her pain wasn't psychological.

She pleaded with him. "I've been to over thirty doctors. They say it isn't my body; it's my head. You say it isn't my head; it's my body. What am I supposed to do?"

He couldn't offer a solution.

With no help from modern medicine, she turned to faith for relief. She struggled, she prayed, and she persisted. There were good periods and bad periods, each for varying lengths of time. In addition to her fatigue and pain, she also battled brain fog. She stared at the pages of a book but couldn't make sense of them. She struggled to find words, and her memory failed. She raised her girls the best she could, and William stepped in to fill the void left by her illness. She watched other moms file in and out of daycare and school and wondered if she would ever feel like them, feel *normal*. She lived this way for twenty years. *Twenty years.*

By early 2005, she was getting worse by the month. Then a friend gave her a book written by a doctor in Louisiana about chronic fatigue syndrome. Clara read it and decided to make an appointment with the doctor/author to see if he could finally provide some answers. She and William were now living in North Carolina, so they flew to Louisiana and stayed in a hotel while the doctor assessed her.

After a detailed review of her history and a physical exam, the doctor said he thought Clara had Lyme disease. She was shocked. She wasn't an outdoor person. She didn't remember getting bit by a tick or having a bullseye rash. How could it be Lyme?

The doctor said, "I have a questionnaire that I want you to take back to the hotel and read. Any question where your answer is yes, write your name, and we'll review it tomorrow."

Still skeptical, Clara and William went back to the hotel and read through the questionnaire. She laughed at one of the first questions, "Have you ever been diagnosed with transverse myelitis?" When they finished, Clara had put her name next to thirty-eight of the forty questions.

Clara's follow-up blood work from a specialty lab confirmed that she was positive for Lyme. Given the length and complexity of her illness, the Louisiana-based doctor knew he couldn't treat her remotely. He suggested she find a Lyme-literate doctor in North Carolina, which she did. Her new doctor put her on pulsed, broad-spectrum antibiotics, three weeks on and three weeks off. At first, she felt worse, but she eventually improved. About a year after she started treatment, she began to decline. The doctor was confused until she mentioned she had night sweats, which prompted him to test for *Babesia*, a common tick-borne coinfection. She tested positive, and a grueling nine-month course of Mepron, an antiparasitic, was added to her arsenal of medications.

After all the treatment, she felt relief. She was freed from her chronic pain and fatigue and went about living her life. She praises William for his support and love along the way, the support that almost led Russ to fire him.

Although she feels blessed, she still struggles with the fallout from her decades-long battle. She sees an autoimmune specialist for her early-stage scleroderma. She sees a pulmonologist for her bronchiectasis. She sees a cardiologist for decreased function in her aortic, mitral, and bicuspid valves. She doesn't tell these doctors about her history with Lyme because she wants to avoid the judgmental stares and comments she's fielded in the past. She'd love to pursue integrative or functional medicine but can't because her insurance won't cover them. So, she prays, and she perseveres.

Greg

And then there was Greg. Greg was the brother-in-law of my lead software guy, Dave. Dave and I talked about Russ's Lyme diagnosis, and Greg's story came out. I've since connected with Greg's wife, Tamie, to hear their experience firsthand.

Greg's problems started around the year 2000. He was experiencing joint pain, and his neck cracked when he turned it a certain way. Doctors diagnosed him with rheumatoid arthritis and prescribed steroids, but the drugs made him feel worse. Fatigue set in, the aches and pains intensified, and it became harder to keep his self-built computer business running. Lyme disease was getting press in his home state of Maryland, and Greg read an article about the disease and its symptoms. He immediately suspected Lyme was the culprit. Although he never saw a bullseye rash, he had a horse barn and spent a lot of time in the woods.

He returned to the doctor, and they tested him for Lyme three times, including a test on spinal fluid. Each time the result came back negative.

Still convinced that Lyme was his issue, Greg made an appointment with an infectious disease specialist at Johns Hopkins. Based on his medical history, the specialist diagnosed him with Lyme and recommended treatment with antibiotics. Greg felt vindicated that he'd found a doctor who believed what his gut told him to be true, but his excitement was short-lived. Insurance refused to cover the antibiotics because he'd tested negative for Lyme. The doctor recommended a different lab that specialized in Lyme testing, and Greg tested positive and was approved for treatment in 2003.

The doctor started with a two-week course of oral antibiotics, which didn't help. Next, he administered two weeks of IV antibiotics, and Greg's condition improved. Emboldened by their success, the doctor gave him two more weeks of IVs. At the end of this second course, Greg tried to kill himself.

From then on, Greg was a different person. The organized man who'd built a successful business suddenly stopped showing up at work. The dependable dad who was always there for every game or recital was nowhere to be found. The sarcastic and funny personality that had attracted Tamie was replaced by depression and apathy.

He would disappear for days at a time, going on drives that seemed aimless. He heard voices and screamed at the top of his lungs, causing his two fearful young daughters to lock themselves in their bedroom. Then, in the middle of the night, Tamie got a call from a psychiatric hospital in Washington, D.C. Apparently, Greg had stormed the Capitol building and pleaded for their help. He told the security guards that someone on the radio told him to do it. His anxiety and paranoia were all-consuming.

The infectious disease specialist claimed they treated the Lyme and that he didn't need any more antibiotics. Greg's aches and pains disappeared, but he clearly wasn't well. He bounced in and out of psychiatric hospitals. First, doctors diagnosed him as bipolar. Later, they branded him as schizophrenic. Psychiatrists dialed concoctions of medications up and down, but he never found peace.

After five years of turmoil, Greg turned to alcohol and prescription drugs to quiet the voices in his head. He visited different doctors and complained of back pain in order to access his drug of choice, hydrocodone. He used pharmacies all over town to keep from being flagged. Tamie pulled him from the brink of death on multiple occasions, and each time, he was scared and desperate to change his ways. Finally, in 2014, he overdosed. Their high-school-aged daughter found him lifeless on his bed.

The emotional and financial damage left behind was immense. Greg's daughter went to years of therapy for the trauma she endured. Tamie struggled with endless bills and back taxes from Greg's imploded business. She described it as ten years of hell with five years of aftermath.

As I listened to her story, I couldn't help but play Monday morning quarterback. Was the antibiotic treatment not enough to kill the neuro portion of the disease? Maybe the antibiotics didn't effectively cross the blood-brain barrier? Or perhaps they did, but persister cells hung on and won the war? Or did he have an undiagnosed coinfection like *Bartonella*? I read case reports linking *Bartonella* to schizophrenia and saw the impact of the disease on Russ. Did they kill the Lyme only for Bart to rear its ugly head? Or maybe it was something completely different? Another infection or imbalance? Instead of looking for root causes, the doctors treated the symptoms. As a result, these questions would remain unanswered.

* * *

Every story I heard was different. Symptoms varied, as did the way traditional medicine dealt with them. Adryin, Phil, and Dierdre found alternative treatment modalities and got well. Clara also found healing but still suffers from the remnants of her disease. And Greg, well, we definitely didn't want to end up like Greg.

It always bothered me how Lyme could be responsible for so many different types of illness. Fatigue, joint pain, nerve pain, heart disease, seizures, Alzheimer's—they were all so different. How could they be from the same source? Finally, I realized I'd fallen victim to the same type of single problem, single disease thinking that I hated about traditional medicine. Humans weren't a simple system. Sure, we had some successes where a single medication or vaccine thwarted a life-threatening disease, but we'd already picked that low-hanging fruit. The multilayered, tangled branches of chronic disease remained, and simple, mechanistic thinking wasn't enough. Like in engineering, we needed a systems-based approach for the next level of problems. After all, humans were complicated multisystem organisms based upon billions of years of evolution. And at the center of it all was the immune system.

The immune system is often referred to in military terms, waging war against malicious invaders. The reality is a bit less bloodthirsty. The best analogy I've read is from science writer Ed Yong in the book *I Contain Multitudes*. He likens the immune system to a park ranger, carefully controlling which visitors are allowed and which aren't. Humans live in harmony with bacteria, archaea, fungi, protists, phages, and viruses. In fact, scientists estimate that the average human body is inhabited by more bacterial cells than there are human cells and that phages and viruses outnumber human cells by more than an order of magnitude. What a stunning thought. Most of the cells within us aren't actually human. Most cells are only visiting, and it's up to the immune system to decide which of the park squatters are good guys that improve our health or bad guys that take it away.

Borrelia burgdorferi causes Lyme disease in humans, but in ticks, it's a synergistic organism. Ticks infected with borrelial spirochetes have increased fat reserves, are less prone to dehydration, and can take in larger blood meals. As the tick injects spirochetes into a human, the bacteria experience a dramatic temperature increase and pH decrease. As a response, they almost instantaneously alter their genomic structure, clipping out segments and weaving in other segments. They continue this recombination over the course of the infection, changing their outer protein coat to help evade the immune system's defenses. If the immune system is robust, it will likely figure out that it's being hustled. If not, then the *Borrelia* sets up camp and gathers provisions. Most of the nutrients the bacteria need come from collagen and collagen-like substances. They seek this material out and degrade it, making a soup on which to feed. Wherever the tissue degrades, symptoms arise. If it's in the joints, arthritis follows. If it's in the heart, Lyme carditis develops. If it's in the brain or spinal cord, neurological problems emerge. One infection, multiple phenotypes.

Then there's the fact that the majority of Lyme patients have at least one or more tick-borne coinfections. *Babesia, Bartonella, Ehrlichia, Mycoplasma, Anaplasma*—the list goes on. Untreated, these infections fester and add to the assault on the immune system. Babesiosis leads to liver problems, anemia, and kidney failure. Bartonellosis leads to encephalopathy, seizures, and other central nervous system disorders. Again, it goes on. Even progressive doctors who test for Lyme don't often test for these hitchhikers that compound the problem.

But the complexity of the disease doesn't stop there. The immune system is trained to respond to the tissue damage caused by each infection. It sends dendritic cells to scout the area and return to ranger headquarters with intelligence. These dendritic cells may return with a protein fragment from the invader, but the damage is so great it may also return with a piece of the damaged tissue. If it presents a piece of self-tissue to the B-cells back at headquarters (a.k.a. the lymph node), then antibody production is triggered. Once that happens, the host has antibodies to self-tissue or autoimmune. The body attacks itself, and more inflammation occurs.

Park rangers are now on high alert, and resources are being consumed on multiple fronts. An opportunistic virus, parasite, or fungus arrives. Typically, the immune system dispatches the invader, but instead, it goes unnoticed due to other distractions. These infections propagate and aggravate the situation. The park rangers work overtime but can't keep up. Chronic inflammation puts hormonal secretions off balance, feedback loops push into overdrive, and immune barriers break down.

Suddenly, there's a tipping point. Illness overcomes the host, but which illness? Which autoimmune disease was triggered? Which opportunistic infections propagated? Which hormone systems got disrupted? Which tick-borne coinfections took hold? And in which tissue did the infection originate?

Add that to underlying conditions like diabetes, obesity, exposure to toxins, genetic predispositions, and more, and you have a smorgasbord of illnesses. No wonder doctors can't unravel it in a fifteen-minute visit.

How could they? Most of the diseases controversially associated with Lyme had no known cause. They were either autoimmune diseases or diseases triggered by immune dysfunction. Well, why couldn't Lyme be one of the reasons it became dysfunctional? Maybe not the only reason, but a key reason for a significant percentage of patients. Recast under this more in-depth framework, it makes sense.

But how do we prove it? Obviously, we need some sort of test to tell us if *Borrelia* is there or not. But what if the gold standard test is flawed? What if it searched for antibodies to the disease? Antibodies are an indicator that the immune system found the invader and developed a robust response. But what if that isn't the case? What if the immune system has gone haywire and the bacteria has successfully evaded and survived? That is, after all, what it's programmed to do. So, there aren't enough antibodies to trigger a lab test, and thus, the patient isn't infected. It can't be Lyme. If you call it Lyme, you're crazy because chronic Lyme doesn't exist, right?

The more I learned, the less I realized I knew.

16

Men with Laser Green Eyes

August - November 2018

Dr. Parker stared at the results. "I have to say, I've only seen levels this high one other time in my career, and he was a range officer at Fort Bragg."

As he looked up, he read the shock in my face and preempted my questions.

"I know it's confusing since your first heavy metals test wasn't so high. But remember, we used a chelating agent this time. It binds to metals and draws them out of blood and tissues. It's a better assessment of the true body burden. Russ's lead level is a problem. I assume this is from his shooting."

I looked at Russ and nodded. It had to be. I wondered if it was the actual shooting, the reloading, or both.

"He also has a dangerously high mercury level," Dr. Parker continued. "That could be from eating lots of fish, or it could be from dental work. You can get the dental work checked to see if it's a contributing factor, and I would avoid large fish like tuna and swordfish. Do you eat that a lot?"

"Not lately. We did in California, but the fish here isn't nearly as good, so we don't eat it now," I replied.

"Well, we already have him on natural chelators like chlorella and charcoal, but with these levels, we need to do chemical chelation as well. We can start with CaEDTA IVs, and then if his dental work checks out okay, we can add DMPS to help with the Mercury. We can do one treatment a week, but periodically, we'll also need to do a mineral IV to make sure we aren't depleting the metals his body needs."

This conversation had happened months ago, but lately, it looped in my head. I was starting to realize that heavy metals might be more important regarding Russ than I initially thought. I was so focused on Lyme and Bart that I didn't truly appreciate these metals' toxicity.

Of course, I knew not to let my kids eat lead paint, but why was lead so dangerous? How did it impact the body? As I started digging, I realized lead mimics calcium and gets stored in bone. The constant remodeling of bone tissue releases it back into the bloodstream, where it unleashes all sorts of damage. Lead competes with calcium to hinder the signaling of neurons, often leading to cell death and, eventually, loss of memory, executive functioning, and motor skills. It promotes blood vessel narrowing and increases blood pressure. Despite all of his exercise and a great diet, Russ was diagnosed with high blood pressure in his mid-forties. Was lead the culprit? Was this yet another symptom we missed?

And mercury was as harmful. Studies linked mercury to neurological problems during development, and scientists were also linking it to the pathological changes associated with Alzheimer's. It upset the nervous system through multiple mechanisms like protein inhibition, disruption of mitochondrial function, increased oxidative damage, and disruption of neurotransmitters. Each new article brought a new catastrophic pathway to ponder. Once mercury was in the brain, it led to depression, paranoia, irritability, hallucinations, memory loss, tremors, fatigue, and more. We could kill off the Lyme and *Bartonella*, and Russ still wouldn't be well.

My fear heightened with every article I read. But my interest in heavy metals wasn't spawned by research papers or by Dr. Parker's comments. It was spawned by my new hatred of Thursdays because Thursdays were chelation days.

It started with mood swings. Russ was calm and pleasant before the treatment, but as soon as it ended, he was manic. Someone stole his keys. Someone left his truck door open. The kids were "little assholes." He yelled. He threw things across the room. Every Thursday afternoon was a dreaded shitshow that settled out by Friday. Even during his good weeks, I still saw the trend. He'd pass out on the couch after treatment and go straight to bed when the kids got home. One Friday in August, things settled out, but they were never quite the same.

I was exhausted from our Thursday routine, so I decided to take the afternoon off to hang out with Russ. We sat on the back deck, enjoying the quiet before the kids got home. Our conversations were awkward because Russ often misused words or drifted topics in mid-sentence. I did my best to fill in the blanks or shift the conversation to something else, but it often felt like a swing and a miss. We'd chat for a while and then sit in silence. He was tired of talking, and I was tired of pretending to make sense of it, so we sat, staring into the depths of the woods. We hadn't spoken in almost ten minutes when I noticed his stare intensify.

"What are you looking at?" I asked.

"You see that tree down by the stream?"

I looked. There were dozens of trees by the stream. After all, it was the freaking woods. I'd gotten used to checking my sarcasm, so I reworded the thoughts in my head.

"I'm not sure which one you mean."

"See the tree that fell? To the left of it."

I looked again. I wasn't sure I was looking at the right tree, but I also wasn't sure it mattered, so I went with it. "Yeah, okay. What about it?"

"Right behind it on the ground, there's a guy dressed in camo. He's spying on us."

Now, he had my attention. I scanned the downed tree and everything nearby. I saw lots of trees, a couple of squirrels, and a plastic bottle I needed to pick up, but no man.

"I don't see him. Are you sure?"

"Absolutely. Go get my glasses."

"Your glasses?" I asked, confused. He used glasses to read but not for distance. "You mean your binoculars?"

"Yeah, yeah. Those. Go get them . . . please."

I smiled at the please. I was trying to get the kids to say it and found myself constantly reminding them. At least someone was listening.

I found his high-end Swarovski binoculars in his closet and brought them out to the deck.

"Is he still there?" I asked.

"Yes. See where that squirrel is? Look at the tree right behind it on the other side of the stream. He's right behind there on the ground."

I found the squirrel and then moved the binoculars back to the tree in question. I then scanned the ground behind it. All I saw was a stump. I lifted my head from the binoculars and focused my eyes on the same area. Still, a stump. But curious, I studied the stump more. It was contoured like the front half of a person lying prone. There was a rounded section that looked like a hat. Knots on the side resembled a face. It was a stretch, but I saw it. Like a pirate ship or teddy bear hiding in a puffy cloud, my imagination turned the object to life.

"Russ, that's just a cool-looking stump. Here, take the binoculars. You look."

He adjusted them for his eyes and then searched. "Huh, you're right. That's weird."

"I'm going to ask Dr. P. if he's been slipping magic mushrooms into your med matrix without me knowing it," I laughed.

Russ laughed but never took his gaze off the woods. We settled back into silence as I picked up my phone and put an entry in my log.

Over the next month, Russ's visual creativity became more frequent. A four-foot stump from a broken tree became a lady. A log on the ground became a sniper. Our landscapers removed these trespassers from the yard, but new ones popped up to replace them. Most of the time, Russ was calm about our new squatters. He watched them from the porch, wondering what they would do next. A few times, he went into the woods to confront them, but this caused them to run off. The whole thing was more of an oddity than an issue. That is, until Hurricane Florence.

It was mid-September, and Florence brewed in the Atlantic right off the Carolina coast. I first saw it on the news while talking on the phone with my mom.

"You have to be freaking kidding me," I blurted.

"What? Is everything okay?" My mom tended to worry and jump to the worst possible conclusions. I used to tease her about it, but my life lately proved her more right than wrong.

"There is a hurricane headed right to North Carolina. It could be a Category 4 by the time it gets here. What a mess."

"Did you ever get the generator installed?" she asked.

The generator. The generator was *supposed* to be installed when we built the house, but the builder imploded as the market crashed and never finished the job. We thought about installing it after the fact, but we had a portable generator, and Russ knew how to back feed it from the panel in the detached garage. It was highly illegal and dangerous, but he was an electrical engineer and knew what to do. Of course, I did not, and electrocution wasn't on my shortlist of the best ways to die.

"No. You know, last week I prioritized house projects, and that was the top of the list. We lose power too often around here. I even called two companies to get quotes, but I still haven't heard back. I guess I'm not going to hear from them for months now. The last time there was a hurricane like this around here, people lost power for two weeks."

The thought of two weeks stuck in the house with no power and two kids, two dogs, and Russ made me want to lock myself in the bathroom until it was all over. These days, life was hard enough, so why not throw in a natural disaster as icing on the cake.

Mom sensed my exasperation. "It'll be okay. The weather people are usually wrong, so maybe it won't be so bad."

I let out a deep sigh. "Seriously, Mom. What karma god did I piss off? My life is getting ridiculous. Is a little break here or there too much to ask?"

For the next couple of days, I stocked up on food and ice. I charged the flashlights and pulled out the oil lamps. I put all of the yard furniture in the detached garage. I skipped Russ's chelation treatment to avoid the excitement that would bring. We hunkered down, but I couldn't say I was ready.

We lost power for the first time on Thursday night. The storm was a slow mover, and it was supposed to last all weekend. Fortunately, it was only a Category 1, and the worst of it was south of us. Still, I figured we were down until Monday or Tuesday, best case. Surely, they wouldn't send crews out in this mess. To my surprise, the power came back on around 3:00 a.m. The next two days, the power went off and on again two more times. I couldn't believe how fast the crews responded.

Then, of course, there were the kids. I'd been concerned that they'd get restless, be scared, and drive me crazy. But they were fabulous. They entertained themselves. They read books. We played board games. I even made up a project for us: Pick your Power. We sat in the basement and wrote all the circuits for the house on pieces of paper. Then we decided which circuits we needed to power with the generator. We made three piles: must-haves, don't needs, and maybes. What better time to do research, right? The kids loved it. They debated whether it was better to power the lights in their bathroom or the basement TV. Not surprisingly, Ryan chose the TV. Then I told him he was responsible for cleaning the bathroom once the power went back on. His aim wasn't all that good with lights; imagine without lights.

"Bathroom, bathroom!" they both yelled.

So, Florence wasn't that bad. The kids were great. But Russ—Russ was a fucking disaster.

As the storm approached on Thursday, his anxiety brewed. He was the disaster preparedness guy. It was his job to think through the top twenty things that could go wrong and thwart them all. He was great at it and had an answer and gadget for everything. But he had to rely on me now, and his incessant pacing wasn't the vote of confidence I needed. I tried to calm him down, but it seemed futile. He moved from room to room as if his energy could divert catastrophe. After fifteen thousand steps around the first floor, he fell asleep in the bedroom chair. Exhausted, I went upstairs to sleep with the kids in case they woke scared in the middle of the night. It was, after all, their first major storm.

Friday morning, Russ woke up irritable and restless. Before we finished breakfast, he was outside mowing the lawn. The landscapers had mowed it a few days ago, but that didn't deter him. There he was, pacing back and forth with the mower in the middle of a freaking hurricane. If the neighbors didn't already think we were nuts, this would tip them off.

The control freak in me wanted to run outside and scream at him. "Why in the world are you mowing the lawn *now*? Stop it before you hurt yourself!" Every ounce of me wanted to get him inside. But he hated how I always corrected him. The storm wasn't that bad, and he was in the front yard where no trees were likely to fall on him. *Pick your battles, Nicole. Pick your battles.* So, I squashed every instinct in my body and let him mow while I headed downstairs to watch TV with the kids. *Enjoy the power while we have it.*

Later, the power went out again. Ryan was waging a massive Lego battle, and I was doing a puzzle with Hailey. I saw Russ walk by the basement window. In his hands was a shotgun.

Guns were a way of life for Russ. They were his favorite hobby, but they were also his security blanket. Russ grew up in constant fear of his older brother, never knowing what torment he would unleash. As a result, both Russ and his younger brother, Doug, developed deep defense mechanisms. Threats were ever-present, and they had to prepare. Doug studied martial arts and became a fourth-degree black belt. Russ developed a love for firearms. Guns were so much a part of Russ that I had no idea how I would take them away.

I'd been thinking about it for months. If Russ continued to decline, it was inevitable. When he had a bad day, I'd obsess in planning. Then he had a good day, and I hoped to avoid the entire topic. But over the last month, with the snipers lurking in the woods, I started the process of removing his access to guns. I convinced him that I was organizing and started shuttling guns to the new safe I installed in the basement. I cataloged everything, trying to remember what he owned. It seemed ridiculous not to know, but he had so many. Some were for concealed carry, some were for competition, and some were merely to have. They were always his thing, and I never needed to keep tabs until now.

I had all the pistols and rifles safely locked away, and he didn't know the combination. Most of our shotguns were for sporting clays, and he never pulled them out around the house. I hadn't gotten to that safe yet because he used it every day for his binoculars, keys, and watch. I was trying to do things gradually. As I saw him storming around the yard with a shotgun in hand, I immediately regretted that decision. Before I called him inside, I went to the safe and changed the combination.

As I finished, he stormed into the garage, soaking wet with the shotgun still clutched in his hands.

"What's going on?" I asked, trying to stay calm.

He screamed. "Those guys are out there! I told you they'd be a problem. Now, there's a new guy with a machine gun. He taunted me the whole time I was outside. We need to call the cops."

"Wow, okay. You . . . You're pretty wet. Let me help you get your coat off."

"Are you not hearing me? There's a guy outside with a machine gun, and you're worried about my coat? You never get it."

I tried to figure out how to respond.

"I'm sorry, but you're drenched. I want to make sure you don't get sick. Do you want me to go out there with you?"

"No, I want to call the damn cops."

"Okay. Why don't you give me the gun, and I'll go get my phone?"

"I'm not giving you a damn thing. You'll take it away like you do everything else! You never get it. There's a man outside right now who is going to kill us! He was on a vine, swinging from the trees and taunting me."

I took a second to process his words.

"A vine? That doesn't even make sense. Why would someone be swinging from the trees with a gun in the middle of a hurricane? Are you sure it wasn't something else? Remember that log that you thought was a sniper?"

The look of hate on his face told me that correcting him wasn't the right move.

"Yeah, that's right. It's always me who's screwed up. I'm the stupid one. You're the smart one. This is ridiculous. Where are the keys to my truck? I'm out of here."

He stormed over to the safe to get his keys. He pulled the combination from his pocket, but it didn't work. He tried it again and again. It didn't open. Only a series of beeps letting him know he wasn't getting in.

"What did you do? Did you do this?" His eyes pierced through my skin.

Tears rolled down my face.

"Russ, you're scaring me. This isn't like you, and you're scaring me. Can I please have the gun?"

"You want the damn gun? Here, have it! I'm done. You can protect this place on your own."

I took the gun from him and stashed it away in the safe.

I hoped the battle was over, but of course, I wasn't that lucky. For the next hour, he belittled me and screamed at me. I took everything away from him—his guns, his money, his life. I trapped him in this house surrounded by threats, and he couldn't do a damn thing about it.

I tried to explain why I was concerned. In all this time, I'd never seen him do anything unsafe with the guns. But this was unsafe. We had kids.

"You want to call the cops? They could take all the guns away from us if they saw you like this."

But he was adamant. I was the problem. I didn't get it. I stopped fighting and took beating after verbal beating.

He eventually tired of repeating the same arguments and paused. He looked at me with pure anguish on his face.

"If you won't give me a gun to defend this place, will you at least give me a gun so I can kill myself?"

As soon as he said the words, I broke down. All the anger, all the fear, all the pain, it rushed out in tears instead of words. When he saw me collapsed on the garage floor, the switch flipped. He calmed down, sat on the floor, and held me.

We sat there while I let it all out. Ironically, as I started to feel better, the power came back on. I collected myself and thought of the kids. What were they doing? Had they heard any of this? We went inside, and all was calm. Hailey had passed out on the couch, and Ryan fell asleep in his room. They didn't sleep well with the storm raging all night, so they crashed. I felt like crashing too, but I figured I'd make dinner while we still had power.

The rest of the storm was uneventful. Saturday, Russ played with the kids. He saw the woman in the backyard, but she was all right. He would leave her alone. Were things back to normal? I wasn't sure I even knew what normal was anymore.

After the hurricane passed, I reached out to Dr. Parker to get his thoughts on the men living in the backyard. I was convinced they were triggered by the chelation treatment, or at least as convinced as I could be when there were a thousand variables in the equation.

Doctors were terrible at designing experiments. *Something's not working. Great, let's change these eight supplements and see what happens.* Then the next visit, they asked if one of the eight made a difference. How the hell did I know? I had thirty pages of notes, and I couldn't tell what the heck was happening anymore. Russ was on buckets of pills and powders, and they changed every appointment. The engineer in me was so frustrated. I couldn't decipher much from my notes, but at least one thing seemed clear. Bad things happened after chelation.

The other emerging trend was that antibiotics made him worse. Back in the summer, I dreaded going off antibiotics. All of his worst symptoms rushed back, and I was on 24-7 damage control. Now, he seemed better *off* antibiotics, and he never seemed to stabilize when on them. He was more irritable, depressed, and fatigued. My research hadn't convinced me that long-term antibiotics were the way to go, and my recent readings on the microbiome cast even more doubt on that strategy. We had trillions of bacteria and other microorganisms living in our bodies. When this ecosystem got out of balance, the implications could be disastrous. Emerging studies linked gut health to depression, autism, Alzheimer's, and more. I wondered if the continued napalm blasts to his gut were making things worse. Was there a gentler approach? He had a massive reaction to the herb tinctures, and we continued to ramp his dose. Could we focus on that and rebuild his immune system through supplements and stem cells? Surely, six months on antibiotics was a good start, and we could use other therapies to help finish the battle?

A long list of questions sat in my lap as I waited in Dr. Parker's office. We'd become friends with most of the staff, and the woman who ran the front desk fit us in on a canceled appointment. I scheduled Russ for a mineral IV treatment, so I could talk to Dr. P. privately. It felt like a critical juncture, and I didn't want to dance around the point to spare his feelings.

We met in his office rather than an exam room. I sat on a couch so low, I wondered if I'd be able to get out. About a year ago, I was in the best shape of my life. I worked out every day and finally hit my goal of doing ten unassisted chin-ups. But other than walking with Russ and the dogs, I hadn't worked out in months. I sunk into the couch and figured I'd enjoy it while I could.

Dr. Parker came in and got down to business. "Well, it seems like things have been pretty rough lately."

"Definitely. The hallucinations have changed everything. Russ's anxiety is at a whole different level."

"I called in a prescription for Xanax after your first email. Have you tried that?"

"Yeah, a few times. It knocks him out. He becomes a total zombie. I give it to him when he's worked up, but I don't want to give it to him all the time because he looks so vacant."

"You can try using a half dose and see if that helps."

"Okay. That will help me control him, but it won't help him get better. What do you think we should do?"

"Well, I consulted with a couple of different colleagues on his case. I think our next best move is to switch to a *Babesia* protocol. We've been hitting the *Borrelia* and *Bartonella* pretty hard, but *Babesia* could be a huge contributor, and our treatment for that so far has been weak."

"*Babesia*? But we took the herbs for that and went all the way to twenty-five drops, and he had zero reaction. I'm not convinced that's a big issue for him."

"You tried one set of herbs for *Babesia*, but there are others. Also, sometimes the herbs have a big impact, and other times, they don't. It could still be what's holding him back."

It didn't sit well with me. "Even if you're right, I know a bit about the *Babesia* protocol from my sister-in-law. You use the anti-malaria drugs, right?"

He confirmed that he did, and I went on.

"That stuff nearly killed her. It tore up her gut. She got bacterial overgrowth in her small intestine, started having seizures, and had massive noise and light sensitivity. It was horrible. And she was *way* healthier than Russ. I don't think he'll make it through the treatment."

"Everyone reacts differently, but I think this is our next move."

He seemed confident, but I was far from it. Every text from Jodi swirled through my brain. The inflammation, the panic attacks, the pain. Russ couldn't take it.

"What about the chelation? I checked my notes, and he's done a total of seventeen treatments. Is that enough to get his heavy metals down? Can we take a break or at least remeasure?"

He shook his head. "Unfortunately, for someone like Russ, he'll probably need to double that to get him to a good space."

"Double!" My jaw hit the floor. I wanted to end the Thursday madness, not have another six months. If we doubled the number of treatments, Russ would end up in the psych ward.

"Yes, double. We can remeasure and see where he is, but I wouldn't expect a huge improvement. It's a very non-linear curve. Usually, patients hit an inflection point where things turn for the better, but it's hard to predict where that is."

We talked over the options until Russ finished his IV. Dr. Parker agreed to let Russ recover a bit before proceeding. We would keep going with herbs, detox, and immune support but would take a break from chelation and antibiotics and see how he responded. I could tell that he disagreed, but everything in my body said that the *Babesia* treatment was the wrong move. I lost more of him every day, and that treatment felt like the final push into the abyss. I left the appointment more disheartened than ever.

The next month was a roller coaster. Some days, Russ was calm and happy, and others, he was frantic. One day, I spent an entire afternoon looking for his binoculars. He was sure that he left them in the trunk of his truck, which he had done—yesterday. He'd probably moved them six times since then, but now they were gone. Better yet, the people in the backyard came in and stole them. Their mischief started to extend inside the house to explain the unexpected or the lost. The Bluetooth tracker attached to his binoculars must have been out of battery because it didn't respond, leaving me to search for them the old-fashioned way.

I looked in all the familiar places: the truck, the closets, his office, the garage. Nothing. Finally, I found them behind a row of books on his office shelf. I wondered what else he stashed in odd places.

Then, of course, there were the people. We hadn't had another day like during Florence, but Russ became increasingly obsessed with our yard guests. With his guns now confiscated, he focused on more creative ways to keep them away. Apparently, chopping down branches from trees pissed them off. He tried to get his chainsaw going, but I quickly sabotaged that pursuit by removing the spark plug. Instead of turning to a manual saw, he hacked at limbs with his hunting knife. Some days, he toiled for hours with only a small pile of limbs to show for his efforts. Loud noises also upset the people enough to make them leave. The times he wasn't chopping, Russ was out with the blower or the weed whacker shooing them away. Going after a sniper with a weed whacker—Lord, help us both.

I tried not to leave Russ alone, but sometimes, I didn't have a choice. One particular day, I had a doctor's appointment for Ryan. Ryan did terrific at the end of Brain Balance, but I noticed his behavior flaring again by the end of the summer. He had bouts of diarrhea and other weird issues with his gut. It seemed like when his gut flared, his behavior flared along with it. I reached out to Rebecca from Brain Balance to get her advice, and she recommended a functional immunologist in Chapel Hill, Dr. Frazier. He had saved her son from the terrible after-effects of a mysterious virus, and he was known for solving tough cases.

After our first visit, Dr. Frazier ran a series of tests. The results were eye-opening. Ryan's zonulin levels were elevated, showing that the thin barrier separating the lumen of his intestines from the rest of his body was broken down. Put more simply, he had a leaky gut. This leakiness caused food particles to penetrate the tissues surrounding the intestines, causing inflammation and a host of food sensitivities. His blood work showed antibodies to almost everything on the panel: gluten, egg, soy, corn, tomato, cacao, dairy, peanut, and yeast. The only thing on the test that he wasn't sensitive to was cod. Yay, cod! He also had latent viral infections and other high inflammatory markers. All the time I spent focused on Russ, I never figured that Ryan also had issues. His ADD was genetic, or so I thought. But what came first, the chicken or the egg sensitivity? Was his gut the root cause of all his problems?

We'd been seeing Dr. Frazier for a few months, and Ryan was already better. His gut stabilized, he wasn't getting in trouble at school, and his grades were excellent. Of course, we completely changed our diet—again—but I was used to that. First, we changed our diet for Russ, then for Brain Balance, and now for Ryan's sensitivities. I carefully selected every item that went in the pantry, and all our meals were homemade. It would be great to call out for pizza, but by then I knew that every single ingredient in the pizza would kill my son. Another skill added to my resume—full-time paleo chef.

Between travel time and the actual appointment with Dr. Frazier, Ryan and I were gone for about two hours. As I stepped out of his office to pay the bill, I noticed six texts and three voicemails on my phone, all from neighbors. *What in the world?*

I called my neighbor, Tom. He and Russ got along well, and his was the last voicemail on my phone. I didn't even listen to his message; I just dialed. I skipped the pleasantries and got right to the point.

"Tom, what's going on?"

"Well, apparently Russ got upset and was walking around the neighborhood with a hunting knife. He ran into our new neighbor and told her that someone broke into his house and killed one of his dogs. She called the cops."

"The cops? And what about the dogs? Are they okay? Did something happen to them?" I never thought Russ would become violent, but maybe I was wrong. *I swear if he hurt one of those dogs...*

"The dogs are fine, don't worry. I was at home and saw the cop car drive by with lights on, so I followed him. He was talking to Russ, and I went over to help out. We haven't talked about it, but I know he hasn't been quite right."

I wondered what he did know. Russ often went on bike rides or walks around the neighborhood on his own, and he loved to strike up conversations. I had no idea what he would share about our little slice of chaos, but I decided a while ago that it was what it was.

"I'm sorry we haven't been in touch. Life's been a bit insane. Last year Russ was diagnosed with dementia. We think the cause is some tick-borne illnesses and heavy metal toxicity, and he's been under treatment since the beginning of the year. Lately, it hasn't been going well."

"I'm so sorry, Nicole. But everything is okay here now. We came to the house and checked it out, and there are no signs of anyone being here. I convinced the cop that all was good, and I've been hanging out with Russ until I could get in touch with you."

"Thank you so much, Tom. I swear I've only been gone for about two hours, and I had no idea this would happen. I took Ryan to a doctor's appointment, but we're on our way home now. I should be there in twenty minutes."

"No problem, take your time." He then added, "You know, I'm about to have time off from work in a couple of weeks. If you want me to hang out with Russ so you can get a break, I'd be happy to do it."

My first reaction to offers for help was always no. I could handle it, and I didn't want to be a burden on anyone. But clearly, I couldn't handle it anymore. Clearly, I needed help.

"Tom, that would be great. If you don't mind, I think I'll take you up on that."

"Please do. Just let me know."

As I hung up the phone, Ryan stared at me from the rearview mirror.

"Is Dad okay? Are the dogs okay?" he asked.

I focused on his innocent little eyes.

"Dad and the dogs are fine. It sounds like he got a little freaked out while we were gone, but he's all right now. Mr. Tom is there with him."

I thought back through my half of the conversation and tried to hear it through his ears. He knew Daddy saw people who didn't exist in the yard. I did my best to shelter him from the worst of it, but you couldn't live in our house and not know. Were his gut issues the results of living in what was becoming an insane asylum? Or were they triggered by the constant antibiotics for his chronic ear infections as a baby? Or both? Yet another unknown to torture my late-night mind.

"Was it the people again?" he asked.

Hearing it out of his mouth felt like an eighth-round sucker punch.

"Yes. I think he got scared, and he freaked out a neighbor. But everything's fine, so don't worry."

When we got home, I let Ryan watch a little extra TV in the basement while I checked on Russ. I thanked Tom profusely and hugged both dogs, relieved that my fear didn't come true. After Tom went home, I made Russ a late lunch. He'd refused to eat all morning, and I'm sure that didn't help anything. We sat on the couch in the living room while he ate.

"So, what the hell happened?" I asked.

"It was those guys. Once you left, they were all over the yard. I was on the porch, and they stared at me with their laser green eyes. When I came back inside, the dog was dead. I didn't know what to do, so I went next door and rang the doorbell, but no one answered. Then I took a walk and saw a woman, and she called the cops."

"What did the cop do?"

"He put me in the back of his car, but then Tom came, and we all came back here. The cop was a great guy. He told me to let him know if I saw anyone again."

I took a deep breath and tried to figure out how to respond. Should I go along with Russ's fantasy story, or should I try and get him to see reality? I'd done both in the past with an equal hit rate of mild success and miserable failure. He seemed calm, so I decided to go with reality.

"Russ, you scared me. I was only gone for a short period, and it got pretty bad pretty fast."

"I know. I was scared too."

"I'm sure you were, and I'm sorry I wasn't here. But remember, sometimes you're sure you see something, and then we pull out the binoculars, and it isn't what you thought. Like the woman in the yard. We looked that time, and it only was a broken tree with a funky knot in it. I think sometimes your brain plays tricks on you."

He got a little annoyed but was still calm. "Nikki, I know what I saw . . ."

"I know you think you saw it, but you may want to consider that you're going through a lot right now. Maybe things aren't exactly the way you think you see them."

He seemed to be listening and taking it in, so I pushed my luck.

"Don't you think it's odd that no one else can see these guys? I can't, the kids can't, Doug was here last month, and he couldn't. It might be your brain messing with you and not anything or anyone else."

He sat there, staring at the coffee table. I wasn't sure what was going on in his head, but I figured I should stop after such an emotional day.

Finally, he let out a deep breath and said, "You know, if I'm that screwed up and none of this is real, then it's time for me to go. This isn't working—for any of us."

He was right; it wasn't working. But I knew the implications behind his words. There was no escape to Atlanta. There was only one real solution in his mind. Every other time he brought it up, my heart ached in dissonance. We could fight; we could rebuild. We could put out the fires and map new routes in his brain. Sure, that could work if the fire was the size of Rhode Island, or maybe even the Midwest. But lately, the whole country was on fire with no signs of easing. Perhaps he was right. Maybe his solution was more humane for everyone.

But what could I do? Give him a gun? Give him a bottle of pills? I couldn't do that. There were so many ways it could go wrong, and even if it went right, I couldn't live with myself. I looked at Russ, and the despair in his face was paralyzing. I loved him, and he was suffering. So, I did the only thing I could think of at the moment. For the first time in my life, I made a promise I had no idea how to keep.

"Russ, don't do that. We aren't there yet. We still have more fight left in us, and we aren't there yet. I know what you don't want, and I promise I won't let it get there."

"You do? Are you sure?"

"I am. Don't worry. I'm strong, and I'm stubborn. We will figure this out, and I won't let it get there."

He looked me in the eyes and smiled.

Later that night, when everyone was asleep, I sat on the back deck to figure out what to do. I analyzed the events of the day over and over again. After about an hour and a full glass of wine, I came to three decisions.

First, I would never leave him alone in the house again, ever. If that meant I had to get help, then that meant I had to get help.

Second, I was going to ask Dr. Frazier to consult on his case. I never made important decisions at work without getting at least three different opinions. Our next moves in treatment were going to make or break him, and I needed more input.

Third, to survive, I needed an end in sight. I couldn't keep doing this indefinitely. I couldn't do that to Russ, to me, or to the kids. I decided to give treatment six more months. If he wasn't on a path to a better place after six months, then he would have to move to a home. It would be breaking the promise I made only hours ago, but I couldn't see any other way.

As I finished the last sip of wine from my glass, I noticed something in the woods. A series of green lights cut through the darkness. We had a neighbor on the back edge of our property, and it looked like part of a security system. *Men with laser green eyes.* For the first time, I saw them.

17

The Nurse and the Engineer

September 2018 - January 2019

I wanted to be prepared for Russ's first visit with Dr. Frazier, but I was overwhelmed as I thought through our past. At this point, over two years of medical history laid scattered in various files. The information was in cabinets, on the computer, in my email. How could Dr. Frazier make sense of it all? I didn't have time for him to come up the learning curve, so I needed to figure out a way to jump-start the process. It was time to let the engineer take over.

First, I organized my computer and printed the relevant files and emails. Paper piled on the floor as my mind forged a plan. Then I hit the file cabinets. I scrutinized every medical folder and put essential documents in piles. Next, I sat down and wrote. Patient history took at least twenty minutes of the first appointment. After what we'd been through, I wasn't going to improv my way through his complex story. I sat down with my piles of paper and wrote a seven-page summary of our medical journey. Finally, I put it all together. I arranged each pile by date and/or importance and then coalesced them into a three-ring binder with labeled, tabulated sections.

Section 1 - Narrative of Patient History
Section 2 - New Patient Paperwork
Section 3 - Health Care Power of Attorney
Section 4 - Lab Test Results
Section 5 - Doctor's Office Correspondence and Summaries
Section 6 - Supplement and Treatment Schedules

The two-inch binder was full. If I included all the bills, it would double the size.

We spent the bulk of the appointment going through the binder. At the end, Dr. Frazier suggested we pull together a team. He would help on the immunological side, but he didn't know enough about tick-borne illnesses. He recommended we include his colleague, Dr. Turner, who practiced in Pennsylvania. Since Dr. Turner was embedded in tick country, he had the needed experience on that front. Next, he recommended a functional neurologist to help exercise and remap Russ's brain. Dr. Frazier knew Dr. Daniels, the same person Rebecca recommended months ago, and he suggested that we work with her. We needed to get Russ stabilized first, but brain exercises would be a crucial part of the rebuilding process. Finally, there was Dr. Peters. He was a local MD with whom Dr. Frazier often collaborated, and his office could help with any infusions or IV treatments. It sounded expensive, but we were in the final throws of the race and losing was not an option.

I spent the next month filling out new patient forms and Fed-exing three-ring binders. The hardest person to get in touch with was Dr. Turner. His calendar booked out for months, and I wasn't sure how to get the access I needed. I was losing hope until I spoke to his medical assistant on the phone.

"Yes, Nicole! You're on our radar. I know we can get you in sometime in the next week or so, but he doesn't want me to schedule you until he's read your binder."

My eyes widened. "You mean, Dr. Turner is going to read the whole thing *before* our appointment?"

"Yes, if that works for you, it will be more efficient. We can bill for his time as a records review, and then your appointment can focus on questions and next steps."

"That's perfect." I made a mental note to ask for this process with any future doctor. If they weren't willing to do it, it was probably a sign that I wasn't in the right place.

When I finally got Dr. Turner on the phone, he laughed a little bit.

"You know," he said, "In all the years I've been practicing, I've only gotten a binder like this from one other patient."

"Really?" I said, a little surprised. "With all the tough cases you see, I figured there would be more."

"Nope, you're the second."

I pondered his comment. "Well, here's an important question. The first binder, did that patient get well?"

"Yes. As a matter of fact, they did," he replied.

"Excellent. Well then, here's to the power of the three-ring binder."

The new team of doctors worked out a plan. We would treat the tick-borne infections with herbals and a few targeted antibiotics. We would also rebuild his immune system, using supplements to support his body's ability to fight off the infection. Finally, we would optimize key markers for brain health that were critical to restoring a regenerative environment. This last piece came from the work of Dr. Dale Bredesen at UCLA. I read some of his papers after Russ was diagnosed with Alzheimer's, but I'd put it to the side after his Lyme diagnosis.

I asked about chelation and whether we should continue those treatments. Everyone on the team was against it. Dr. Frazier called chemical chelation dangerous and likened it to a flirtatious partner at a dance. Yes, it was good at drawing people out onto the dance floor, but halfway through the dance, it let its partner go and grabbed another one. The newly abandoned was now mobile and angry. Who knew where it would wander to spread damage? Chelation would more likely make things worse. We would use supplements to grab whatever mobilized naturally, but we shouldn't force cranky partners onto the dance floor. *Great. Russ only had seventeen cranky dance parties. What damage did that do?*

As I reviewed our new supplement and treatment strategy, I should have felt relief. I now had a team of doctors saying what my gut told me for months. So, why was anxiety still running the controls in my head? How did I know if these doctors would get it right? How much damage did I do with the previous one? I thought he was good until suddenly, I didn't. One doctor said chelation was the way, and the other said it was dangerous. One put him on Xanax, and the other said it worsened his dementia. I spent five years studying semiconductors and was a fledgling in immunology. How the hell was I supposed to figure this out? Russ wasted away neuron by neuron while I clamored to get my shit together. I couldn't learn fast enough to keep up, and every new thing I learned called into question everything I thought I knew. The responsibility felt like a massive vice cranking tighter on my chest.

Meanwhile, while I waged a twelve-round boxing match with my conscience, Russ focused his battle on the woods. Every chance he got, he obsessed about the people. He wasn't seeing them, which I guess was good, but he *knew* they were up to all sorts of mischief at night. Piles of tree limb clippings emerged each morning as evidence of their presence. In reality, it was the forgotten damage his hunting knife had made the day before.

He went on and on and on. He couldn't let it go. I tried to be calm and go along with it for a bit and then cleverly divert him. It worked for a while, but he got right back to it. I played defense all day and by the time night rolled around, I was exhausted. Then one night, as I prepared for the kids to get home, he shared his grand plan.

"I know what we can do!"

The energy in his eyes concerned me right from the beginning.

"Tonight, after the kids go to bed, we can go out there in that thing. You know the camo one?"

I stumbled to fill in the blanks. I was getting pretty good at it. "You mean the deer blind?"

"Yeah, that thing! We can put it outside and sit in it. You can have the rifle with you, and then when we see them, you can shoot them."

I couldn't believe what I heard. This was his grand plan? He wanted me to sit outside in the middle of the night in thirty-degree weather clutching a rifle waiting for people that didn't exist. *Are you fucking kidding me?*

It was the last straw. I screamed at the top of my lungs.

"Russ, there's no one in the backyard! Nothing but squirrels and some damn deer! Will you please stop obsessing about shit that doesn't exist? I have enough to worry about with the things that are *real!*"

Predictably, he got angry and stormed off. I heard his truck door slam, but I'd disconnected the battery, so I knew he wasn't going anywhere. By the time I followed him to the garage, he was already gone on his bike.

The kids came home, and Russ ignored us for the night. Our only contact was a note he left in my closet.

"I've pissed off the queen bee, and I'm not sure why. I will be leaving and going to Atlanta soon."

Damn it, Nicole. This isn't working. You're living the definition of insanity. Think differently. How are you going to solve the problem?

I sat in silence for a while. Then, it came to me in two simple words: sensor net. I could build a sensor network in the backyard. If I placed devices on trees, I could link them to an app on my phone to alert me anytime someone was in the area. We could do it together as a project, and maybe it would give him the feeling of protection he needed.

The next day I talked to him about the idea, and he seemed to like it. He came up with issues, but his logic was long gone, so I quickly argued them away. He seemed excited to have a new answer to his growing problem.

The engineer in me got to work. I researched sensors and cameras and scoped out mechanical parts. As I planned out Wi-Fi boosters and app connectivity, I realized the insanity had rubbed off.

Okay, back off, MacGyver. You don't need to custom design anything, and this doesn't actually have to work. I don't want an alarm going off in the middle of the night when a deer family scurries through the yard. Keep it simple and make it look credible.

I diverted my search to Amazon and purchased a set of motion-sensor activated lights that looked like cameras. I planned to mount them to trees and use photos and a mocked-up screenshot to convince him we were wired. I felt guilty for lying to him, but if it brought me some peace from the people, then I would gladly take my time in purgatory.

A few days later, my Amazon packages arrived, and it was time to do the install. The kids were at school, my morning was clear of meetings, and it was a beautiful fall day. The plan was going perfectly until I remembered that in my life, plans no longer mattered.

Russ stormed into the kitchen while I sorted boxes and parts. The look on his face threw a familiar tightness across my shoulders, and I braced for the storm. I attempted to divert the onslaught.

"Hey, are you ready to install the new security system with me?"

His stare let me know I'd only taunted the lightning.

"What? I don't give a shit about that. Do you know why my truck doesn't work? I need to get out of here, and my damn truck doesn't work. Nothing ever works around this place!"

There were different levels of his anxiety, and I could tell we were on DEFCON 2, high alert. It wasn't going to be the morning I'd planned.

"Don't worry; we'll figure it out. It's probably the battery again."

I knew exactly why the truck wasn't working. It was hard enough to contain him around the house. I didn't need to extend my plight to the state of North Carolina.

My calm demeanor amplified his anger. It was clear he wanted me as frantic as he was.

"I'm telling you this is a *problem*. Every time I want to go somewhere, that thing *never* works. We need to get the damn thing fixed."

I looked around the kitchen and noticed his breakfast still sitting on the counter. He always seemed more agitated in the morning. So much so that I brought it up in our appointment with Dr. Frazier, who noted it was probably his blood sugar levels. The disease damaged glucose metabolism pathways in his brain, and his neurons were starving for fuel. Blood sugar was lowest in the morning, and the result was a case of the hangries on steroids. I needed to get him to eat.

"It's fine. We can jump it and go for a ride. Why don't you eat something first, though?"

"I don't want food. I want my damn truck! You always do this! You're the one that traps me in this damn house with no guns surrounded by people who want to *kill* us. First, you take my money, then you take my guns, and now you take the damn truck. It's ridiculous!"

Deep breaths. DEFCON 2 meant he argued. It didn't matter what it was, it was wrong. It didn't matter what I said, it was stupid. If argument were a sport, he'd take home the gold.

I tried to figure out how to turn the tide. Dr. Turner recommended exogenous ketones to help feed his brain. We'd done MCT and coconut oil to provide ketones when he was first diagnosed with Alzheimer's, but I'd let it fall to the wayside in all the mess of supplements. The ketones Dr. Turner recommended had high BHBs or beta-Hydroxybutyrate levels, which readily circulated through the body and crossed the blood-brain barrier. I grabbed the new container from the pantry and mixed a scoop in a glass of water while attempting to calm Russ down.

"The truck is fine, and I have the security system that we talked about right here to help with the people in the back. I was hoping you could help me with it today, so we can get it up and running. Here, have a drink. It tastes like lemonade."

He fought like a cranky toddler. "I don't want food, lemonade, or anything! Stop trying to give me stuff. All I want is to fix my truck!"

"Okay, fine. Then hold this for a second. I need to get these boxes sorted, and then we'll go check it out."

It was a trick I'd learned from a nurse at Dr. Parker's office. Tell him to take something, and he wouldn't do it. Ask him to hold it, and habit would bring it to his lips without him realizing it. Sure enough, a few seconds later, he started to drink, and the sweetness compelled him to keep going until it was gone. I'd hoped it would be a bridge to get him to eat something. Instead, something more dramatic unfolded before my eyes.

Within minutes, his tone softened, and the constant shouting ceased. His muscles, clenched and ready for battle, surrendered one by one. His shoulders relaxed and hung comfortably in their rightful place, and his hands, formerly fists, spread out and gently touched the countertop. The intensity in his eyes diminished, and a hint of sweetness emerged. It was like Mr. Hyde was tamed, and Dr. Jekyll reemerged.

I was stunned by the transformation. One drink couldn't have an impact so quickly, could it? Eager to understand the new person standing in front of me, I probed.

"Are you okay?"

He looked at me and flashed a tender smile. "Yes, I'm good. I was thinking about how lucky I am to have you."

He grabbed my hand across the kitchen island and held it as he walked around until he was next to me. He put his arms around me and held me tight.

"I love you. I know sometimes I'm a jerk, but I want you to know I love you."

I hugged him back despite my bewilderment. A few moments ago, I was the shrew who stole all of his earthly possessions, but now I was his love. What the hell happened? I knew we were all a collection of chemicals and signaling pathways, but I'd never imagined that the biochemistry soup controlled the show. We had free will. We could control how we acted and reacted, right? What I witnessed was a clear vote for biochemistry as the real power.

He leaned back to look at me and placed his hands on my cheeks. Tears formed in his eyes.

"I don't know where I'd be without you," he said.

He kissed me and then resumed his embrace, this time holding me even tighter. I melted into his arms. I wasn't sure what happened, but it had been a while since he held me. I let my confusion go and realized how much I needed that comfort.

After watching the impact of ketones on Russ, I started giving him half doses every two to three hours. The results were astonishing. The sweet, caring man I fell in love with replaced the constant anxiety that plagued the previous months. While the kids were at school, we went for long walks and bike rides. I took him on errands, no longer worried he would storm out of the store. While I worked, he played the guitar. I made a CD of all of his favorite songs and put it on a repeating loop. Sometimes, he'd play for hours on his own. Other times, he would stop and check on me. Most of the time, I'd lead him right back to playing as if it was a new activity for the day.

He still saw the people in the back, but "sensor net" was working. He'd find something suspicious in the yard and claim it as evidence. Then, I picked up my phone and investigated.

"Nope, no alerts. Camera shots are all clear. Oh, here's a photo of a deer family from 3:00 a.m. The buck probably made that rub mark with his antlers."

It was all manufactured with stored images, but he felt protected and safe. And apparently, my little project seemed realistic because even my neighbor noticed and asked if I would recommend the installation company. *Umm, no, definitely not.*

Life went on like this through the New Year. As long as Russ drank his ketones, he was good. If he got his dose too late or put it down without drinking, it was an instant shitshow. I usually saw it coming. He paced back and forth, looking for something but unsure what. Then he got irritable. The slightest comment or noise made him tense. Finally, he exploded. Some event or lost item pushed him over the edge, and all the nastiness flooded back, only to subside as soon as he got his dose. Sometimes, it was a matter of minutes. Other times, it was three to four hours in hell trying every trick to get him to drink.

I'd reached out to home aide companies before but never pulled the trigger. He was so unstable. I wasn't sure anyone else could handle it. When Doug visited in the fall, I asked him to watch Russ for a few hours, so I could go to an important meeting at work. By the time I got back, Doug looked more frazzled than a new dad with quadruplets.

"I have absolutely no idea how you do that every day," he said. "It's only been three hours, and I feel like I'm insane."

I envisioned helper after helper quitting, each time dashing my hopes for even a moment of sanity. But now he was calm, and he was manageable. So, I reached out to Visiting Angels, and we hired Amy.

Amy was a Chinese woman in her early fifties. She was a hard worker, extremely reliable, and very sociable. Russ got along with her pretty well, at least most of the time. Every few visits would be a bit rough, and he referred to her as the "crazy lady that follows me around." I was glad that she replaced me as the "crazy lady" since, on multiple occasions, he mentioned the "crazy lady that looks like you." I laughed because I figured his description was more right than wrong.

For me, Amy was a lifesaver. I got out of the house on my own for the first time in months. I went back to the office and met with people in person instead of endless video calls. I volunteered to chaperone field trips and to be a lunch parent at school. Little things I used to take for granted became novel and revitalizing.

I also started reading and researching again. When I initially went part time at work, I planned to use the extra time to study and manage Russ's treatment. Over time, my role morphed into a constant caregiver, and there was no time for research. I longed to learn, to help, to stay ahead. Instead, I merely reacted. If we were going to get through this, I needed to be more than a caregiver. I needed to be a nurse working hand in hand with the doctors to get him better. I needed more knowledge, more training.

I poured myself back into Dr. Bredesen's work. It was a core part of Russ's treatment, and I already saw the massive benefits of mild ketosis, one of the program's core tenets. I read his books, watched lectures on YouTube, and read research papers. As I assimilated everything I learned, I realized my entire framework for Russ's disease was wrong.

For over a year, I ran away from an Alzheimer's diagnosis. And who wouldn't? Alzheimer's was the kiss of death. Accepting it meant accepting a horrible disease with no cure. It meant piles of useless prescriptions and nearly a hundred billion dollars spent on failed trial after failed trial. Russ didn't have Alzheimer's. He had Lyme, *Bartonella*, *Babesia*, and heavy metal toxicity. Those diseases were treatable, and Alzheimer's wasn't.

But Dr. Bredesen shifted the framework. Alzheimer's wasn't a disease; it was a symptom. The brain was constantly remodeling itself as part of everyday life. Synapses that got used were reinforced, and those that didn't were broken down and built into different memories. It explained why, despite three engineering degrees, I could barely remember any calculus. The process was natural and governed by a protein called APP or amyloid precursor protein. If APP got cleaved by proteases into two pieces, it led to blastic, or building activity that supported memory formation and maintenance. If APP got cleaved into four pieces, it led to clastic, or destructive activity that led to the loss of synapses. In Alzheimer's, the balance was tipped toward the clastic side so that destruction reigned. In fact, one of the four pieces in the clastic APP reaction was the amyloid-beta that became synonymous with the disease.

But what caused the imbalance in the first place? Fortunately, nature was smart enough not to put one thing in charge. That would be too dangerous and easily corruptible. Research showed at least thirty-six different contributors deeply embedded in cardiovascular, metabolic, hormonal, and immune system health. Alzheimer's wasn't a cause; it was an effect. A downstream symptom of a problem or multiple problems that existed upstream. It was akin to a fever. A fever wasn't a disease. It was a symptom caused by an infection. The trick was, which infection? Was it pneumonia, sepsis, or the flu? The key to understanding Alzheimer's wasn't treating it like some fabled disease with a magic pill. It was figuring out what caused the symptom in the first place and addressing the root cause.

It made perfect sense. It explained why we had a family friend who slowly declined over twenty years, while Russ dropped faster than a rock in a quarry. According to Dr. Bredesen, there were different causes and even types of Alzheimer's. Type 1 patients suffered from chronic inflammation. Type 2 patients had suboptimal levels of hormones, nutrients, or growth factors. Russ was type 3, characterized by exposure to toxins, such as heavy metals, mycotoxins from mold, or tick-related toxins from Lyme and Lyme coinfections. Lucky us, he had two of the three.

So, I was wrong when I said Russ didn't have Alzheimer's; instead, he had Lyme, *Bartonella*, *Babesia*, and heavy metal toxicity. In actuality, he had Alzheimer's *caused* by Lyme, *Bartonella*, *Babesia*, and heavy metal toxicity. The root cause was vital and something the Alzheimer's community was so desperately missing.

The Bredesen program outlined lifestyle changes and supplements that could turn the tide and once again tip the balance back toward the building side of the equation. It was everything I'd come to believe about optimizing health. Managing diet, exercise, sleep patterns, hormones, stress—a holistic approach that influenced all of our biochemical pathways. His research team had not only prevented but also *reversed* dementia. It was monumental.

But as I read on, I realized subtleties mattered. Dr. Bredesen's approach was the least effective for Type 3 patients. With Type 3, it was critical to address the toxins and infections first. I was trying, but destruction still reigned, and Russ's cognitive skills continued to fail.

Still, we persisted. We did three more stem cell treatments. Each treatment brought a small improvement, but those improvements quickly faded. Dr. Turner recommended an experimental treatment with high doses of Dapsone. A leading Lyme doctor saw great results with hard-to-treat patients. Again, positive changes, but no restorative balance. We stepped up his dose of natural chelators to pull out circulating metals. There was no noticeable impact. The map was still on fire. I was losing more of him every day and beginning to lose myself in the process.

18

The Banshee

February 2019

Russ came down to the basement gym looking for me. "What are you doing?" he asked.

"I'm trying to squeeze in a workout," I answered. "I'm so out of shape these days. I need thirty minutes, and I'll be back upstairs. Why don't you go play the guitar?"

"Good idea," he said.

He turned, and I heard footsteps climbing the stairs. Soft thumps echoed above as he paced in the living room. Five minutes later, he was back.

"What are you doing?" he asked again.

"I'm trying to work out. I have about twenty-five minutes left. Is it okay if I finish? I need this to work off the crazies."

It was true. I didn't even feel like myself anymore. I felt like a more uptight, high-strung version of me, and that was saying something.

"Of course. I'll be in the garage."

Again, he walked off. Again, he was back in five minutes.

"What are you doing?"

My jaw clenched. I tried to think of a different approach.

"I'm working out. Do you want to join me?"

"No, I'll let you finish. How long will you be?"

"About twenty more minutes. The time is right there on the screen." I pointed to the video I was following. "Is there something wrong?"

"Not really. I was just looking for you."

He stood there staring, watching as I did each push-up, each burpee. I kept going. I needed this workout. Eventually, he wandered off. He came back at seventeen minutes, at eleven minutes, at eight minutes. As he hovered during my cool down, I realized the workout hadn't cleansed the crazies as I'd hoped. I felt tenser, more annoyed.

It was mid-February, and each day was about the same. I was the Pied Piper, and wherever I went, Russ and two little dogs followed. At first, it was nice. Russ was mostly relaxed and amiable, and spending time with him brought me joy. But it didn't take long for me to feel cramped. I needed a little time every day to recharge, to fill my cup. That time never came. When Amy was at the house, I was off to work. There, I dealt with issue after issue, trying to squeeze forty hours worth of work and influence into half the time. Then, I came home, and Russ was always there, waiting and watching.

His need for constant companionship made it hard to spend time with the kids. He was calm around me, but the kids had too much energy and were too loud for him. Whenever they came around, the same pattern emerged. The kids entered the room and inevitably started fighting. Hailey, being younger, lost the fight and screamed or cried. The noise agitated Russ, and he got angry and irritable. I played damage control to contain the situation. I shuttled the kids to the basement to watch TV. I pawned them off on playdates. Entire weekends passed without even thirty minutes to focus on them.

When I met Russ, his independence had captivated me. On weekends, if he had nothing to do, he went out on his own. In the winter, he packed up his gear and went skiing. In the other seasons, he went hunting, shooting, fishing, or mountain biking. Unencumbered by other people, he went off and made friends along the way if he felt the need for company. Later in our marriage, his independence often served as a frustration. I needed help with the kids, but he spent all day in the yard. I wanted quality time, but he focused on a new rifle reloading recipe. Now, I longed for even a smidgen of that independence to return. Thirty minutes to take a bath, a walk, a workout, a nap, anything.

Later in the day, I made an early dinner for Russ and me. Ryan had basketball practice at 6:00 p.m., and Pauline would feed the kids and meet us there. For two years, I'd been Ryan's head coach. Basketball was always my favorite sport, and watching him grow to love the game was my dream. I couldn't choose his hobbies, but I could expose him and see what stuck. Fortunately, basketball stuck perfectly. This year, I knew I couldn't be the head coach. Russ was too unpredictable. So, I let Ryan go through the draft, and when his coach reached out, I offered my services as an assistant. She was the only female coach in the league and welcomed the help. It was kismet.

I prepped Russ all afternoon for the evening ahead. Usually, he watched from the sidelines or went outside the gym, where it was quieter. Basketball wasn't his thing, but he often enjoyed watching us play. As I cleaned up dinner, I went over the plan again since it was almost time to leave.

"So, after I finish the dishes, I'm going to grab my sneakers, and we'll head to basketball practice, okay?"

"Practice? I don't want to go to practice. Can't I stay here?"

I knew that wasn't a good idea. Five minutes after I left, he'd panic and head over to the neighbors' house.

"No, I want you to come. Ryan loves having you there. Plus, I need you to keep an eye on Hailey."

A little white lie. Hailey was always fine at practice. She read a book or played on her tablet. I was less worried about her at age five than I was about Russ.

He continued his protest. "Why didn't you tell me this earlier? I wanted to sit and relax a bit."

"I did tell you earlier, and we'll relax when we get home. It's only an hour."

"An hour, ugh! You go, and I'll be fine here."

I felt the snapping turtle rising within me. We needed to be on the road in five minutes, and this wasn't going well.

"Come on, babe. I need your help with Hailey at practice. Please, you said you would."

"How about I take my truck, and then I can leave if I need to? I can even take Hailey."

Ugh. That was a worse idea. There was no way he was driving the truck or Hailey anywhere. It would be a perfect plan if everything was normal, but we passed normal a long time ago. We were six snipers and a vine-swinging Rambo past normal. I tried to stay calm. Four minutes.

"It's not that long, and there's no gas in your truck. Plus, Ryan likes to talk to you after practice. I promise it'll go fast."

Russ argued. "Why can't I stay here? Why won't you let me take my truck? Why do I need to be there at all?"

With each volley, I got snippier and snippier. Two minutes.

I grabbed my bag and moved to the garage to change the scenery. Russ stood next to his truck and argued. He looked for his keys. One minute.

I raised my voice, and he got defensive. "Why are you yelling at me?" Zero minutes.

"We have to leave. Please get in the car. I can't go without you."

He didn't understand. One minute late.

Frustration rose like a tidal wave. All I wanted was to coach my little boy, but I couldn't get him in the damn car.

"Just get in the damn car!" Two minutes late.

"Why are you yelling at me? Why are you so angry? I didn't do anything," he kept repeating it. Three minutes late.

"Argh! *Please* get in the *damn car*! We have kids, and they need me too! I want to do this for Ryan."

I felt the tears coming, building. He still didn't understand. Four minutes late. I really hated being late.

"Fine, I'll go. Help me find the keys to my truck. I'll follow you there."

Even breathing didn't help. He pleaded for his keys. Five minutes late. I had Ryan's shorts because he forgot them. He'd have to practice in his school uniform pants. He was waiting. Now, he'd be late. *Why couldn't I get him in the car??*

"Please, Russ. Please, please, please, get in the car. I'm begging."

"What's wrong with you? Why are you acting this way?"

"Why am I acting this way? Why am *I* acting this way? All I want is to go and coach our son in basketball. That's all I want. I give and give and give to everyone. But this is important to *me*! I want to be there. I want to go!"

"Then go!"

"Ahh! You are ruining my life!"

The tidal wave crashed. I stormed into the house and slammed every door between me and the bedroom. Tears weren't enough. They didn't express the anger, the pain, the grief. I threw my bag across the room and screamed. I screamed like a banshee crying in the night. I wailed as if letting it out would release the demon growing inside me. I screamed again and again and again.

With all of the anger released, only despair remained. I sat down and cried. Russ came in and tried to console me, but I was too far gone. Overuse broke my reset button. I wanted to leave this house, to raise my kids, to maybe sleep for a little while.

Russ started talking about leaving, about going to Atlanta. I began my standard defense to the common discussion, but then I realized he wasn't trying to escape. He wasn't imagining a better life for him somewhere else. He was imagining a better life for *me*—one without him in it. He was trying to make *me* stop hurting. I looked at his face, and he was crying, destroyed by the fiasco happening in his brain.

His tears reminded me of how sick he was. They reminded me that it wasn't his fault, that he couldn't control the confusion and turmoil occurring in his head. I held him while we both wept. I'd been a terrible caretaker that day. The desperation in his sobs made me understand why my tears always turned him around. It shifted perspective. It triggered new emotions. I saw life through his eyes—and it was scary.

19

Plan B

April 2019

When I was a kid, Easter was my favorite holiday. It was the one big holiday where we didn't pack up all our stuff, jam ourselves in a car and go for a tortuous, all-day car ride to someone else's house. Easter was *our* holiday, and everyone came to *our* house. I even got to stay in my bed because it was a small twin size where no one wanted to sleep. No one, of course, except me. I had many fond memories of Easter. Family surrounded us, we feasted on succulent dinners, and I watched TV all day while the adults caught up on people I didn't know. It was glorious.

As an adult with my own family, Easter was not such a big deal. A couple of times, my brother and parents came, but the tradition never stuck. Growing up in a dysfunctional family, Russ never felt the need to see family on holidays, and long stints with my family tended to make him edgy, even before he got sick. As social as he was, afternoons on the couch watching sports or movies weren't his thing. Russ needed to tinker, work, or exercise; otherwise, his boundless energy came out as crankiness. Then, of course, the sicker he got, the worse his behavior became.

One year, before Hailey was born, my parents and Scott's family came for the holiday. Other than evenings, Russ was distant for most of their visit. He retreated to the garage, worked in the yard, went to the shooting range, anything to keep himself busy. He came in to shower before dinner and then proceeded to be his jovial, playful self. All was good for a while, but then one dinner, the conversation drifted to guns and politics. Russ was passionate about both and typically argued his point with reams of facts, diffusing any tension with a witty joke. But this conversation, fueled by too much alcohol, got out of hand. Before I knew it, Russ screamed at both Scott and Dad. Tension built and erupted, and Russ stormed out. I was stunned and mortified. This was a family dinner. This was supposed to be fun. What happened?

I hoped that calmer and more sober heads would prevail, but no, Russ stayed angry for two days. He slept in the detached garage and avoided everyone for the rest of the holiday. I couldn't believe how childish he acted. I knew he had anger issues in his twenties and thirties, but I'd never seen them firsthand. Maybe the newlywed bliss wore off, and the true him came through? Or, in hindsight, was it an early sign of his illness triggered by stress and alcohol? I'd never know the actual cause, but the effect was a lonely series of Easters from then on.

Fortunately, we built new traditions. Our neighbors, the Driscolls, were becoming our adopted family, and we decided to plan a fun weekend together. I didn't know how the powers that be decided to deal Russ's illness to our family, but they extended an olive branch when they put the Driscolls around the corner.

Rick and Russ were the first to meet. They were about the same age and hit it off when they realized they were both shooting aficionados. Rick introduced us to the rest of the family, which unexpectedly mirrored ours. Tiffany was younger than Rick and was about my age. They had a son, Tyson, who was Ryan's age, and a daughter, Lindsey, who was Hailey's age. Our unusual little family had a doppelganger. Even more unbelievable was that our families filled with strong-willed individuals *liked* each other. The Driscolls became our best friends and were some of the only people who knew the slice of madness our life had become.

The Saturday before Easter, Amy came over to watch Russ so I could spend some time with the kids. Tiffany planned to take the boys to a trampoline park while I took the girls to a ceramic painting store. Afterward, we'd meet up and take all the kids out to lunch. It was a simple day, but I looked forward to it all week.

Once we settled in at a painting table, the girls and I selected our projects. I picked a ceramic Easter Bunny, Hailey chose a small canister shaped like an apple, and Lindsey went straight for a cute serving dish to make for Tiffany. I loved to do crafts and hoped that some quality time with the girls would relieve my growing stress.

Hailey's project was pretty simple, so she finished first. Lindsey and I were far from done, so I encouraged Hailey to add more detail or grab another project. She painted a little more on her apple but then lost interest.

"Mom, can you come with me to wash my hands?" she asked.

I was immersed in painting, and the sink was only fifteen feet away. "Hailey, you can go by yourself. It's right there."

She lumbered off but came back excited. "Mom! You should see the things they have in the back. They're awesome! Come look with me."

I barely looked up from my second coat. "Hailey, I'm painting. I'll see when I wash up. Why don't you add something fun to your apple?"

"Like what?" The whiny voice started to peek out.

She grunted a bit and painted some polka dots on her apple. Finished for the third time, she played with the paints.

"Hailey, be careful," I said. "You almost knocked Lindsey's water over. Go get another project if you need something to do."

"I don't want to. I'm *booorrred*." There it was, the whiny voice. My jaw clenched and my shoulders tightened.

"Well, Lindsey and I have more to do, so you're going to have to figure something out." I paused and looked around. "Hmmm, where's the blue? I need some blue."

Hailey tried to pass the paint, and a big blob of blue imprinted itself on her sleeve.

"Hailey! Be careful!" I snapped. "You're going to get paint all over your clothes. Go get a paper towel from the sink."

"Can you come with me?" she asked.

"No, it's right there. You can get it."

She dragged her shoes all the way to the sink, and when she came back, she stood next to me. She grabbed my arm and kissed it.

"Hailey! You bumped me while I was painting! Please be careful!"

I shot her a stern look that could peel the paint right off her apple. She put her head down and made her way back to her side of the table. She sat down with her chin hung by her chest. I put down my head and looked at my bunny.

Stupid little bunny. I focused on three coats for this stupid little bunny instead of focusing on my daughter. Doing. I had to keep doing whatever it was. Making dinner, cleaning up, laundry, feeding the dogs. I was *doing* all the time, and I'd forgotten why I was doing in the first place. I looked over at Hailey; her five-year-old head still hung low. I'd yelled at her for kissing me. For kissing me! Who was I? What was I becoming?

I took a deep breath and put the bunny down.

"Hailey, why don't you show me the stuff in the back? I think I need a break."

Her eyes lit up, and she jumped out of her chair. She didn't want a perfectly painted apple or a stupid little bunny. She only wanted some time with her mom. Fortunately, my thick head realized that all I wanted was time with her too.

On Easter Sunday, we planned a big Easter egg hunt at the Driscolls' house. We'd sworn off candy at the beginning of Brain Balance, so on Saturday night Ryan and Hailey helped stuff each egg with little toys and piles of change we gathered from Daddy's coin cup. Ryan put extra quarters in the yellow ones and bragged that he would get them all first. After I shuttled them off to bed, I played the Easter bunny. I planned a treasure hunt with clues leading them to the motherload of gifts, including books, Legos, puzzles, and some fun Easter crafts. Of course, none of it was done, so at 10:30 p.m., I sorted through Amazon boxes, trying to remember what my grand plan even was. I pulled everything together and climbed into bed around midnight.

At 3:14 A.M., Russ woke me up. "Did you hear that?"

"Hear what? No, I didn't hear anything. I was asleep."

"There was a banging noise. I think he's in the house."

Oh crap. Not again. At least two or three nights a week, Russ woke up early, convinced they were in the house. Sometimes, it was a bang as the air conditioner started, and sometimes, it was the crash as the dog door closed. Whatever it was, I knew it wasn't mysterious people with green eyes.

"It's probably house noises. The alarm is on, so there's no way anything is getting in."

"I'm sure I heard something. I'm going to check it out." He pushed up on his arm to get out of bed.

"Wait, let me check my phone." First, I went to the system that worked.

"Look, the security cameras, they're all fine. No motion alerts for the last six hours." Next, it was time to go to my fabulous concoction in the backyard. "Nothing in the back either. No new photos from an alert. Let me check the house and the kids, and I'll be back. You stay here."

I left the bedroom and shut the door. Usually, by the time I got back, he was sound asleep. I then drifted in and out of crappy sleep patterns until the alarm went off at 6:00 a.m. This night was no different. By 4:00 a.m., he was dead to the world, and there I was, exhausted but still awake.

The next morning, the kids immersed themselves in their Easter spoils, and Russ looked through photo albums in his office. Even though I was tired, I decided to take advantage of the situation and squeeze in a quick workout. I was showering when Russ paced his way into the bathroom. As soon as I saw his eyes, I knew. *Shit. I forgot his morning ketones.*

The next hour was filled with pacing, yelling, and pleading. It was almost time to go to the Driscolls, and Russ was still frantic. I scrambled to get ready as I begged him over and over again to drink. As I followed him into the garage, ketones in hand, I saw Ryan.

"Mom, I'm ready. Can I ride my bike over to the Driscolls?" he asked.

"No," I blurted back. "We'll all go together in a little bit."

"Mom, why can't I go? I'm ready, and I want to see what they got for Easter."

"Ryan, I said no! Chill out and wait. We'll be ready in a bit."

As I finished talking, I tripped on Hailey's shoes and spilled the ketones all over the place. The shoes I'd told her thousands of times to put on the shoe rack and not in the middle of the floor. I picked them up and threw them across the garage.

"God dammit! Why doesn't anyone listen to me in this damn house!"

Ryan stared at me in shock. His lips quivered, and he started crying. He ran into the minivan, screaming, "I didn't do anything! I didn't do anything!"

Remorse flooded over me. Ryan hadn't done anything. I chewed his head off for wanting to ride his bike to his friend's house. I followed him to the minivan and put my arms around him.

"Ryan, I'm so sorry. You're right. You didn't do anything. I didn't want you to take your bike because it's supposed to rain in a little bit. But I didn't say that. Instead, I snapped at you. I've had a rough morning with Dad, and I didn't mean to take it out on you."

"I didn't do anything," he muffled through his tears.

"I know. It wasn't your fault. It was mine. I tell you what, let's get calmed down, and then you can ride over to the Driscolls. Just be sure to put your bike in the garage. If it rains, we can leave it there, or I'll throw it in the minivan. I'm so sorry. I was so focused on Dad, I . . . I couldn't think clearly."

After Ryan headed off, I went back to the bedroom and collapsed into what was becoming my crying chair.

Russ walked in and came over to console me. I took advantage of his compassion and went to the kitchen to give him a full scoop of ketones. I wanted to avert a crisis for the rest of the morning. Fifteen minutes later, he was fine, and the three of us drove the short distance to the Driscolls in the minivan.

The Easter egg hunt was wonderful. The kids scurried around the yard, screeching and laughing, all trying to outdo each other with their next find. Russ laughed and joked around with Rick. This was my life. Beautiful moments separated from complete despair, sometimes by only a matter of minutes.

Tiffany saw the look in my eyes. "Are you okay?" she asked.

"I'm tired, Tiffany. I'm so tired."

That night, while the kids settled in to watch a movie and Russ retreated to the bedroom, I sought the solace of the back porch to relax and unwind. I thought back over my weekend, my year, my life.

My life was filled with accomplishments. In high school, I was valedictorian and captain of four teams: soccer, basketball, tennis, and math. At MIT, I earned a perfect GPA and was captain of the basketball team my senior year. In my career, I threw myself into industries I knew nothing about, and within months, I earned the most complex assignments. I was a vice president at a growing, high-profile med-tech company before the age of forty. I married my best friend. I had two beautiful children. Success after success after success. But as I sat there on the deck evaluating my life, all I felt was failure.

At work, I'd spent the previous week preparing for a portfolio review. I crafted each slide deck with the project teams, and we thought we were ready. Then I reviewed the materials with my boss, and it seemed like everything we did was wrong. I was the one who bridged expectation gaps. I was the one who pulled everyone on the same page. Now, I was a hamster on a wheel throwing away a week's worth of work. There was no progress, no value-added. There was only motion.

Then there were the kids. Ryan talked about his Tae Kwon Do teacher at dinner, and I had no idea who she was.

"I've had her for a while now," he said. "Ms. Pauline knows her."

Yes, your sitter knew her, but I didn't. The last time I sat down and played with them seemed like a distant memory. Lego and robotics sets from Christmas sat in the corner, waiting for a free hour of my time. When they were home, I barked at them for no reason. I jumped on every mistake to avoid triggering Russ. Often, he wasn't even that bad. It felt more like me. I was more stressed, more emotional. I was constantly on alert.

And then there was Russ, still struggling in almost every way. We finished brain camp with the functional neurologist the week before. I knew it wouldn't bring back the man I married, but I hoped for maybe a little sliver of him. He seemed more engaged and happier the weekend afterward. His sex drive was back, and we rediscovered for the hundredth time how much intimacy helped both of us. But then he faded. His interest in me waned. His mood slipped into apathy. Most importantly, I couldn't see a single inkling of improved cognitive function.

Things were also getting more insane around the house. Russ used glue remover to clean the kitchen counters. He came into the house with a small branch with twisty little twigs and said they were wires that electrocuted people. I chuckled, finally understanding what he was talking about for a few days, but later broke down when I pondered the absurdity of his thinking. Then one night, as I locked up the house, I found urine all over the pantry floor. The sheer volume told me it wasn't the dogs, but I still couldn't believe it. As I cleaned on my hands and knees, I grappled with reality. Was this the future? Where was the intelligent, fun-loving, ultra-competent man I married?

The only thing left that felt like him was the guitar. He played beautifully, and it brought him peace and comfort. But even in that silver lining, I noticed holes. A missed note here or a string out of tune there served as a harbinger of abilities wasting away. All the research and the time and the money, and I still failed. I failed miserably. The man who was my partner and my soul and my love was slipping away. All my successes meant nothing because I failed at the one thing that mattered most. The pain felt like a thick cloud suffocating me.

I looked through the window and saw the kids snuggled up in their blankets as they watched the movie. A conversation with a close friend flashed into my head. Her dad had a debilitating stroke when we were in elementary school, and she spent most of her childhood with a sick parent. When Russ was first diagnosed with Alzheimer's, I asked her for advice.

She looked me straight in the eyes and said, "Nicole, if you can afford it, put him somewhere that can care for him. Don't let your kids watch their dad die. It was horrible, and I'll never forget it."

It was Plan B. For a long time, I avoided Plan B. I knew it might be a reality. I knew it was a probable outcome, but I didn't need it yet. Then in the fall, when the hallucinations worsened, I asked my mom and dad to look into a place for him. I needed this, but I couldn't be the one to do it. How could I fight the war while also planning retreat?

My parents wanted to help but didn't know how, so I asked them to find a place that could care for him. A nice place where he could be comfortable and happy.

My mom made calls, researched, and narrowed it down to a few facilities in the area. Then, when they were in town for Christmas, in between the festivities, they went to visit "friends." Each visit was a tour where they gathered information and prices. They narrowed the list further, and all that remained was for me to see them and decide.

The thought of getting our lives back seemed like a dream forever out of reach. I longed to leave the house, to have people over, to go on vacation. I wanted to live without playing defense all the time. All my efforts and Russ still declined. He wasn't getting better. But the kids, they were still growing, learning, becoming. *Don't let your kids watch their dad die.*

I decided to get serious about Plan B. I would ask Tiffany to come with me to see places. I wanted someone there to lean on, to help. She was the rock I needed.

I looked ahead to my month at work. I didn't care about anything on my plate. This process was going to be awful. I needed to be focused, to heal, to be there for the kids. It was time to step away from my job.

I needed to figure out what we could afford. We were well off, but resident care was expensive. I had to review my finances and see if we could afford for me to take time off, particularly with enormous new expenses.

Plan B was becoming real.

I kept thinking about the day, the weekend, the future. What would Russ want? I knew what he wanted for himself, and I couldn't give it. I couldn't give him the peace we'd given Radar no matter how much I wanted it. What would he want for us? For me? For the kids? I knew what it was. Plan B had to become Plan A. It was a massive shift that I didn't take lightly, but as hard as it was, it was right.

So, there it was, a new Plan A. My heart was relieved and destroyed at the same time.

20

New Places at the Table

May 2019

I sat in the bathroom, staring at the mirror. I couldn't remember how long it had been since I'd been in the house alone. Months? Years? It was so quiet, so peaceful. I could think.

I dropped Russ off at the Charles House, a wonderful place that cared for dementia patients during the day, so caregivers could rest or work. We'd had a trial visit the week before, and I was a wreck. How would he react to being around other dementia patients? Would everyone else be older? Would he be confused in a new environment? Would he see all the signs that said dementia care and be angry? Then again, maybe it would be good for him. At home, he followed me around all day because he was bored. He needed stimulation, something to do, but he couldn't do that on his own anymore. There was no way I could keep him occupied all day. Maybe their programs and activities would help him.

On the trial day, he entered the room, cautious but confident. The director offered us both a seat at a large oval table filled with new faces and began a round of introductions. There were two facilitators and twelve other patrons. A North Carolina State University professor, an accountant, a nurse, an elementary school teacher—each person had their own story of triumph and loss. The group reviewed the news of the day, which drove a discussion of the events. The facilitator did most of the work, but she drew everyone in with her adept mastery of conversation.

I stayed at the table for about ten minutes, and then the director pulled me away in a prearranged plan to leave Russ on his own. I assured him I'd be back in a bit and then settled into the room next door, watching the group through one-way glass. As I studied Russ with silent anonymity, I was amazed. He sat with a presence that I recognized but had almost forgotten. He listened intently and then commented, causing the entire group to erupt in laughter. He pointed to another person and clapped his hands, giving him accolades for whatever he added to the conversation. He sought eye contact, and his demeanor and charm pulled people in. The words were likely garbled and lacking in wit and sometimes sense, but watching only his body language, I saw the dynamic executive I once knew. He controlled the room, and his smile was contagious.

Russ passed the trial visit with flying colors, and I scheduled him into the only openings they had available, afternoons three days a week. We called it his job, and he was excited about his new colleagues and the work to be done. It was his first day, and I reveled in the strange silence of an empty house.

I thought of the Charles House as a bridge, a test to see how he would react and engage in a group care environment. Trained by history, I, of course, expected the worst. But as I analyzed his interactions through the one-way glass, I realized I was thinking of Russ as he used to be, a fiercely independent man who never liked to show weakness or need. Getting him to open up took years of conversations, trust, and eventually love. But he was a different man now. He needed help, stimulation, guidance, and social connection. Most of all, he needed a sense of self-worth, and a community could give him that. Perhaps moving him to a facility wasn't only the best thing for the kids and me; maybe it was also best for him.

Since Easter, I'd wound down my responsibilities at work and placed Russ on the waitlist for two full-time facilities. Waitlists were usually tortuous disappointments, but this one had a unique agony. I was sitting around, hoping someone would die to make space for him. How freaking awful. Someday, some other desperate family would pray for Russ's death to make space for their loved one. Not directly, of course. There was nothing malicious about any of us. It was the way the process worked.

It was now early May, and a spot at Brookhaven, my first choice, opened up. The facility handled only dementia care patients, and they had several other mobile and active residents like Russ. It was a homey environment, and the staff was friendly and caring. I visited several places, but somehow, I knew that Brookhaven was the one. He could move in at the end of May.

My brain, my heart, and my soul all implored me to say yes. I was broken and exhausted. I'd given so much to Russ's care that I'd lost myself in the process. I needed this. The kids needed it. Even Russ needed it. So, why did it feel like rabid squirrels were eating me alive from the inside? The decision was logical but devastating.

Without interruptions and looming catastrophes ruling my day, my thoughts melded together. I had never grieved. I lost my husband piece by piece, but I never mourned his passing. A few days before, Russ's old work friend reached out to check in on him. I'd never met this friend, but the stories preceded him. The conversation was challenging but lovely, and after we spoke, he sent a text to thank me. At the end of our text exchange, he added, "You know when Russ spoke of you, he always said how lucky he was to have you. He said he didn't know how a dumbass like him got so damn lucky, but he was sure glad he did."

His words hit my raw emotions, and before I knew it, I was bawling on my closet floor. Within minutes, Russ found me and lovingly asked what was wrong. I took a deep breath and shoved the pain down somewhere deep. Deep enough to convince him all was okay. What else could I do? Tell him it was killing me to watch him waste away? Tell him smells of urine and dozens of confused conversations replaced the memories of the real him? Tell him that every hair-brained explanation for a misplaced item made me want to scream? Or should I tell him that I missed my partner, who sometimes knew what I thought before I did? That I missed the person who always listened and who turned my vantage point upside down with one simple sentence. What good would telling him any of that do? It wouldn't snap him out of it and bring back the man he was. It wouldn't cure him of his awful fate. It would make him sadder, more depressed. So, another day passed, and the grief piled up.

Our thirteenth wedding anniversary was only six days away—lucky number thirteen. In thirteen years, my transformation from ecstatically happy to hopelessly miserable was complete. Logically, I'd figured that Russ would pass away before me. We talked about it while we were dating, and I told him, "Well, I would rather have twenty great years with you than forty crappy years with someone else." I figured we had plenty of time. We had time to raise our kids and watch them move out on their own. We had time to finish our tour of sporting clay courses across the country and ski every mountain in the Rockies. But by the time I picked up my head from the mess of bottles and diapers and endless hours of *Sesame Street,* I was already losing him. I thought twenty years was a low bar, but I didn't even get to thirteen.

And despite all the yelling and tears and banshee screams, I still loved Russ. The depth and sweetness in his eyes told me I captivated him as much as that heated night in Japan. As he played the guitar, his body showed the passion that music erupted in his soul. So much was gone, but the remnants peeked through from a time filled with love, laughter, and adventure.

Russ filled my thoughts, and I wondered how he was doing. I picked up the phone and dialed. The director picked up.

"Hey Paul, it's Nicole Bell. I was curious how Russ is doing on his first day?"

"He's doing great. The staff loves him! He already seems to have made a few friends and has everyone laughing. I think he'll fit in perfectly here."

Relief poured over me. "That's fabulous. I wish I put Russ with you all months ago instead of getting someone at the house. It seems like what he needs."

"Don't worry about that. He's here now, and we're happy to have him. You relax, and we'll see you in a few hours."

I hung up the phone and took a deep breath. Maybe I could keep Russ at the Charles House? Could I wait for a full-time slot to open up? But the Charles House wasn't open on nights and weekends, precisely when the kids were home. He'd only get worse. *Don't let your kids watch their dad die.*

I dialed the number for Brookhaven before I lost my will. A newly familiar voice answered.

"Frank Stalman here."

"Hey, Frank. It's Nicole Bell. I've thought about it, and I want to go ahead and reserve that room you have available. I think it's time."

I selected Russ's move date very deliberately—Friday, May 24, the day before my forty-third birthday. All I wanted was to spend my day with the kids, 100 percent focused on them. It was the most messed up birthday present I'd ever given myself, but I wanted it more than anything. One day of predictable happiness, or at least as predictable as it got with a five and eight-year-old.

Over the next two and a half weeks, I spent every spare moment preparing. I ordered furniture and arranged for delivery. I furiously shopped at Homegoods to make his room cozy and comfortable. I filled out endless reams of paperwork, outlining financial status, medical history, likes/dislikes, and daily routine. I packed supplies and clothes and arranged them in his new room. I bought a small Bose radio, so he could play the guitar along with his favorite CDs. Each four-hour slot he was at the Charles House was a flurry of packing, driving, decorating, or whatever task needed completion.

I also tried to prepare Russ for the transition. I wasn't sure if it was more for my benefit than his, but I didn't want to spring the transition upon him. I wanted him to understand, to be ready, so I looked for a window to introduce the idea. There was something inside him that knew things weren't right. He often sought change but didn't know what that looked like or what to do.

In one such moment, I was preparing lunch. Russ walked up and stared at me across the kitchen island.

"You know, I was thinking—this isn't working," he said with a look of desperation on his face.

"What do you mean?" I asked, shifting my attention from our salads to him.

"I don't know. I don't do anything anymore. It doesn't feel right." He was lucid and calm. I realized this was as good a time as any.

"Well, you seem to be enjoying the Charles House. That's going well, right?"

"Yeah, those guys are great. Really smart. I'm glad to help out."

"Well, I've been talking to another place that needs even more help. It's a live-in community, and they want someone to entertain the residents and even help with some maintenance around the property. I think you'd be perfect for it."

Fortunately, Frank had said they often had residents who "worked" on the property. They melded it into their daily activities.

"I met their maintenance guy, and he's ex-Navy," I continued. "You'll love him, and he said he has a list of projects where he needs help. And the activities director said you could play the guitar every day after lunch to entertain the residents. She's super funny, and I think you'll get along great with her too."

"Really? Huh. You think I could do it?"

"I know you can. You'll be perfect. The community needs coverage around the clock, so you'd have to live there, but the good news is, it's close by, and I can visit anytime."

His face looked puzzled. "You mean you wouldn't be with me?"

"Not all the time, but I would be there a lot. Now that I'm not working, I was thinking about volunteering there myself." I saw the concern on his face soften, so I piled on. "Don't worry; you're stuck with me. It would kill me if I didn't get to harass you regularly." I flashed the smile he used to call my shit-eating grin.

He chuckled. "Okay. That sounds good then." He paused, looked me in the eyes, and went on. "You know, I love you more than anything in the world. I hope you know that."

Both of our eyes swelled with tears. "I do . . . and that feeling is mutual."

The morning of the 24th, I was wound so tight I could feel the stress coming out of my pores. I drove the kids to school, intentionally not sharing my plans for their dad. A few nights before, Ryan asked a simple but loaded question, "Mom, what happens if Dad doesn't get better?"

Part of me wanted to foreshadow the events ahead to help him prepare. I tried to be honest with the kids, but I couldn't share my burden with them. They were so young and innocent, and I wanted them to stay that way. It would be awkward for Ryan to live with his dad knowing he'd soon be gone, and I couldn't handle the barrage of questions that would undoubtedly follow.

In the end, I kept my plans to myself and said, "You know, I think about that every day. For now, you let that be my job, and you let your job be doing well in school and setting a good example for your sister."

When I got home from dropping off the kids, I asked Russ to play the guitar. His energy often fed off of mine, and if I didn't relax, the whole day would be a colossal mess. I set him up with his favorite CD and slipped downstairs to meditate in the sauna. I'd bought the sauna for Russ to help him detox through the mess of treatment, but it had become a sanctuary for me. A place I could meditate and breathe, even if only for five minutes. Fortunately, the music mesmerized Russ, so I got twenty minutes of much-needed peace to calm the voices in my head.

Frank and I arranged for Russ to arrive right after lunch. Russ would give a private concert in a small living room outside his new bedroom. They invited a few of the more active residents to watch his performance and meet Russ. Once he settled into playing, I'd leave, and they'd take it from there.

Frank's words echoed in my head. "You know, it's harder for the family members than it is for the residents. We know how to do this, and he'll be fine." I hoped more than anything that he was right.

Everything Russ needed was waiting for him at Brookhaven. My only job was to keep him calm and get him and his guitar supplies in the car around 12:30 p.m. Brookhaven was flexible on timing, so I didn't even have to stress about that. It seemed surreal how relaxed and comfortable they were in the midst of the chaos that came with dementia. A resident got upset, and someone diverted them to a new activity. A full cup of milk splattered all over the floor, and two or three sets of hands swarmed in to clean it up. There was a team of people to keep everything in line, and that team was more effective than any one person could be, more effective than I could be.

Russ and I both showered and then took the dogs for a long walk. By the time we got home, it was almost 11:00 a.m., so I prepared an early lunch. While Russ finished eating, I gathered up his guitar gear. I put the amplifier and his guitar stand in the minivan and then went upstairs to the guest bedroom closet to find the Fender guitar case. Non-sick Russ always preferred to play the Les Paul, but for some reason, sick Russ preferred to play the Fender. It was his lifeline, and I wanted it to be with him as long as he needed it.

I found the case and brought it downstairs, then laid it on the floor and pushed the locks outward to release the latch. The locks didn't move. *Shit. It's locked. Where in the world is the key to this thing?* The guitar hadn't left the house in over ten years. *Shit, shit, shit.* Russ was very particular about his things, and I knew he wouldn't be interested in transporting the guitar without protection. *Okay, calm down. Just find the damn key.* It seemed easy enough. It would have been easy if Russ hadn't been tucking random items in random places for the last twelve months. That tiny key could be anywhere.

As calmly as I could, I asked Russ for his key chain. There was one little key on it, but it wasn't a match. I went out to the safe. On the door, we had rows of keys to who knows what. I grabbed every tiny key I could find. Key after key after key failed to open the case. I searched his closet and his dresser, where he stored random items. Three new keys but none of them were the one I needed. I checked the drawers in his office, nothing. Panic settled in. *All this time planning, running errands, preparing, and now, I get taken out by a tiny little key?*

I took a deep breath. *Okay, Nicole, if you panic, he'll panic. Relax. We have three other guitar cases. See if it will fit in any of those.*

I went upstairs and took inventory. Both the Les Paul and the Martin cases were custom formed to the shape of the guitar. They wouldn't work. But the SG case was a big old rectangle, and it still opened. I walked it downstairs and tried it for size. I had to adjust the foam inserts a bit, but it would work for the short car ride. *Would he notice?* The old Russ needed everything in its proper place, and this guitar wasn't in its proper place.

He walked in as I closed the case. "What's up?"

"I was getting the guitar packed up so we can bring it over to Brookhaven. I can't find the key to the Fender case, so I'm going to use the SG case. It's not a long ride, so it should be fine."

"Oh, okay. Is it time to go?" His nonchalance surprised me.

"Just about," I said. *Relax, Nicole. The other day he asked whose house this was. I doubt he remembers which case goes with which guitar. Relax.* Years of walking on eggshells wore my expectations thin.

We packed up the guitar and a few other odds and ends, and it was time to go. As I watched Russ walk to the minivan, it struck me that this would likely be the last time I ever saw him in the house, in our home. The place we'd designed from a blank piece of paper and had toiled over every selection, every issue, every piece of furniture. I squashed the emotion and kept moving. I had a plan to execute.

At Brookhaven, Frank and I prearranged everything. Frank came out to greet us, so Russ wouldn't realize the front door was locked from both outside and inside. I intentionally stepped in front of the sign that said dementia care, so it wouldn't trigger confusion. Frank gave Russ a tour while I brought in all the equipment and set it up. Sharice, the activities director, came with me to learn how to set up his gear in the future. Then she went to gather the other residents to come and enjoy their private concert.

When Russ walked into the small living room, he smiled. "There's the boss," he said, putting his hand on my shoulder.

Frank was behind him and jumped in. "We had a great tour. I even showed him where he'd be staying while he's helping us out." He ended with a nod in my direction to let me know all was going well.

"Excellent. Are you ready to play?" I asked. "Sharice is getting everyone ready, but we should make sure everything is set up correctly since your roadie kind of sucks."

He laughed and sat down. As he checked the guitar, I threw in his favorite CD. It was Jim Adkins, a smooth jazz artist who almost no one knew. Russ had heard about him in New Hampshire, when his neighbor had given him the CD. The neighbor once lived near Adkins and watched him play in a local venue. The first night Russ listened to this music, it spoke to him, and he spent the entire night playing along. At the time, I lived in Boston, and we were an emerging item. The next morning, I woke up to a five-minute message on my voicemail. It was Russ playing track number nine, "Take Me There." Russ played the lead and added rifts around the melody in a magical way. It brought me to tears. I saved it for months and listened to it over and over again. *Damn, I wish I still had that recording.*

As he started to play, I could tell by his expression that something wasn't right. Did the guitar get knocked out of tune in my makeshift case? Were the amplifier settings wrong for this small room? "What's up, babe? Is everything okay?" I asked.

"No, something doesn't sound right. This isn't going to work."

I feverishly checked all the settings on the amp. Then, I turned up the volume on the Bose. His face relaxed.

"There we go," he said. I laughed at myself—tiptop roadie, capable of adjusting the big volume dial.

The group rolled in, and Frank introduced Russ to everyone. Like the Charles House, Russ controlled the room as if it was his all along. When he was ready to begin, I advanced the CD to number nine. I wanted him to start in his comfort zone. His fingers took off. Frank's eyes lit up as he realized Russ was talented. I guess he didn't know what to expect in this environment. As I moved Russ's things in, I saw that even their paid acts were questionable. But despite his decline, Russ's playing was still world-class.

I watched from the back of the room as Russ captivated the somewhat captive audience. In all my time preparing for Russ to move in, I'd focused on the negatives. The woman in the corner with her head on the table, no matter how many times they adjusted it. The lady who screamed when anyone offered help. The smell of urine or even feces as a resident walked by. I'd gone back to my minivan and cried, realizing that Russ would soon be one of them.

But as I watched the group surrounding Russ, the positives flooded in. The couple who walked arm and arm, offering each other companionship. The activities and outings that kept residents happy and engaged. The hugs and laughter that staff members brought wherever they went. Like at the Charles House, Russ would be okay. It might even be good for him.

After a few songs, Sharice gave me the big eyes and swished her hand at me. "Go!" she mouthed as an enormous, not-so-subtle hint.

I never visualized that part in all my planning—the part where I walked out and left Russ there. I paused to listen a bit more, but Sharice's look let me know I was pushing my luck. Not quite ready, I snuck back to his room and did one final check to make sure all was in place. It was perfect. It looked like a place he could be comfortable. I let out a deep breath, walked past the room filled with my favorite music, and went home.

*　*　*

Ryan busted in the door first. "Hey, Mom! What's for dinner?"

"Your favorite, tacos. It's ready, so go wash your hands."

Hailey and Pauline came in together.

"Do I smell tacos?" Hailey asked. When I nodded, she made a big fist pump to show her excitement.

After Pauline left, the kids gathered around the table, which was fully set.

Ryan was the first to notice. "Wait, what's going on? Why are there only three plates?"

I'd thought it through and prepared. "Well, it's time to switch things up a bit. Before we sit down and eat, let's go to the living room. I want to talk a bit first."

They got quiet and followed me wide-eyed to the living room and sat down.

"I want to talk to you about Dad. I think you both know it's been hard around here lately. Dad hasn't been getting better, and it's been tough on me to make sure he's okay with everything else I need to do. So, today I moved Daddy to a place that can care for him better than I can. They specialize in helping people like Daddy, and they have all sorts of activities and events that will keep him busy and happy. And the best part is that it isn't that far away, so we can visit him anytime we want. He's still your dad, but he'll be living there instead of here."

All expression drained out of Ryan's face as he tried to process my words. "Wait, what? Dad isn't here anymore?"

"No. He'll be staying at a place called Brookhaven. It's a good place for him. They want him to play the guitar for the residents there, and he'll have all sorts of people to interact with. It's kind of like the Charles House, but he'll be there all the time instead of only during the day. And, as I said, we can go see him anytime we want."

Ryan stared at me. Hailey got antsy and looked over her shoulder, eying the dinner table.

I went on. "I think it's going to work out better for everyone. Dad will be happy and cared for, and we can do some of the things we've never been able to before. For example, I thought maybe tomorrow we could go to the mall and go to ZinBurger for my birthday dinner. Then we can walk around and use those gift certificates from Christmas that we haven't been able to spend."

Hailey smiled, but Ryan still looked pensive. "That sounds great, but is Dad okay with it?"

"Yes. Today when I left him, he was playing the guitar for a bunch of new friends. He has his own room, and they feed him all his meals. They have regular outings to restaurants and museums. I think he'll be happier there."

Hailey writhed her body backward, more interested in tacos than the discussion. I took her hint. "Do you guys want to eat? We can talk more over dinner."

At the dinner table, Russ and I usually sat across from each other. Ryan was on my right, and Hailey was at the end of the table on my left. With Russ gone, there was a big gaping hole. A constant reminder that someone was missing.

"Since it doesn't make sense to sit where we used to, I thought we'd move things around. I can sit in Daddy's seat. Hailey, you can sit next to me on my left, and Ryan, you can sit across from me in my old seat. What do you think?"

"How come I don't get to sit next to you?" Ryan asked.

"Well, you get to sit across from me, so you can see my smiling face all through dinner." I flashed the shit-eating grin, and he smiled.

"I think it works. Plus, I'm staaaarving!" Hailey blurted out.

We talked about the day more over dinner. Ryan asked every question that popped in his head about Brookhaven. He asked about the food, the people, Dad's room. He even asked what TV they had.

Then, he remembered the other part of our conversation. "Wait, you mean we can go to the mall tomorrow? And does this mean I can have friends over?"

"Absolutely. It'll be a lot easier for the three of us to do things together. I even thought we could go visit Uncle Scott at his new house in Scottsdale over fall track out."

Scott and Jodi had taken the plunge and built their new life in the desert. The change in environment boosted Jodi's recovery, and she returned to her healthy self. Their new house was a kid's paradise with a pool, a volleyball court, a basketball court, a fire pit, and a batting cage. It even had a private casita where we could stay. I was a bit worried Ryan would defect and join the other half of my family.

Ryan's eyes lit up. "Seriously? That would be *awesome*! I am so in!" He paused for a second, clearly pondering something. "I think this is the best conversation we've ever had at the dinner table. You know, like talking through stuff?"

His innocent words validated all the hard decisions of the past month. "Yeah. I think so too. I'm excited to spend more time together. In fact, let's keep going. How about we stack the dishes in the sink and do them in the morning. Then we'll have enough time for movie night!"

Both kids shrieked in affirmation, and we shuttled down to the basement to watch a movie. The two of them fought over who would snuggle with me. Even my anti-snuggler, Ryan, wanted to get in on the action. We scoped out the movie running time and set a timer, so we could switch halfway through. Holding them and watching them laugh at silly comedy was precisely the birthday gift I needed.

When the movie was over, we made our way up the two flights of stairs to the bedrooms. We were talking about the movie when Hailey spontaneously shouted, "Yay! Daddy doesn't live here anymore!"

Her words brought me to a screeching halt. Ryan saw the look of shock on my face and chastised her.

"Hailey, that's mean. Don't say that," he said.

I pulled myself together and jumped in. "No, it's okay. I know it's been bad around here, particularly for you, Hailey." Hailey's screaming triggered Russ, making her a victim of his bad behavior. "I'm so sorry we all had to go through it, and we can't change that. But we can focus on the future. We'll all do our best to learn and grow and have fun. And we'll make Daddy proud, okay?"

"Okay," they said in unison.

After they went to bed, I sat in the living room in silence. My shoulders, previously tethered to my ears, felt relaxed, back in their rightful place. My back teeth had a gap between them like someone loosened a knot. My body sunk into the chair, deep and loose.

The insanity of the past few months washed over me. I couldn't acknowledge it while I was living it. I had to keep going. I had to be strong. But as the memories of the hallucinations, the anxiety, the screaming, and the crying ran through my mind, I could finally see it, and I had no idea how I'd made it through. I belittled myself for my failure to save Russ, but maybe that wasn't what I was meant to do. Perhaps success was surviving. Getting through safely and sheltering our two little kids as much as I could. I survived, and that in and of itself was an accomplishment.

My journey was far from over. Looking around at the other Brookhaven residents, I wondered which phenotype would afflict Russ. Alzheimer's was his most feared way to die, and all I could do was pray for dignity and peace in the rest of his path. There would be hard times ahead, but if I could keep this house a happy place—a place of comfort and warmth and love—if I could do that, I could get through whatever was next. I survived living amongst the madness, and if I could manage entrenched within, I could undoubtedly manage from afar. Most importantly, shielding and protecting the kids would reap benefits well beyond my years.

Keep this place happy. Build the home Russ and I envisioned.

I could do it, and I felt Russ's spirit with me to help.

21

Who am I?

"Hey, Holly, what's up?" Holly was the executive director at Brookhaven. She was always pleasant and helpful, but getting a call from her still felt like being summoned to the principal's office.

"All is okay. I was just wondering if you're coming here today. I'd like to chat about something."

"I'm on my way now and will be there in about five minutes. Do you want me to stop by your office when I get there?" I asked.

"That would be great. I'll see you in a bit."

I hung up the phone and made the last few turns into the facility, a routine I repeated four to five times a week. My first tour with Tiffany was still fresh in my mind—the smells, the vacant stares, the remnants of life. I'd gone home and cried for over an hour. But being there all the time, I saw the life and happiness that coexisted with the despair.

Residents became friends, and I learned their stories from conversations with them or their family members. Bob and Donna were a married couple who lived together in one of the doubles. Bob had been an attorney and loved Corvettes. Donna was in Brookhaven to be with Bob, and she used her sharp wit to make sure the staff kept everything up to standards. The one thing she couldn't convince them to do was to keep a stash of Honey Bunches of Oats, so she recruited me as her Costco runner. Joseph, Russ's new best friend, was one of the younger residents and a former botanist. His wife Janice was lovely, but caring for Joseph had impacted her health quite severely. As we swapped stories, Janice noted that Joseph also had Lyme. They also had a horrible infestation of mold in their home due to a faulty vent placement. *Hmmm.* Lucy was a scientist and walked in a constant loop around the residence. She never made eye contact or acknowledged my presence unless the kids or the dogs joined me, in which case she became animated. Each of the fifty residents had their story, their family, their loss. The cost of Alzheimer's became more apparent with each new encounter.

Holly's office was the last door on the right before entering one of the resident wings. I knocked, and she invited me in.

"I have to admit that I'm nervous," I said. "You're great and all, but your job typically isn't sharing the good news."

She laughed. "Everything is fine. Russ is doing great. But I did want to tell you that he's been spending a lot of time with Daisy lately."

Daisy was a new resident on Russ's hall. I'd spent several hours with her on the outing to the State Fair and found her very sweet. Despite that, I knew what Holly was insinuating. It was the dirty little secret of memory care, or probably any assisted living. Men were in short supply, and when a new one showed up, there was no shortage of suitors. Of course, they didn't tell me that when I considered placement. I learned it the good old-fashioned hard way.

It didn't take long to figure out the dynamics of the dementia dating scene. My indoctrination occurred during my second visit when I met Priscila. We struck up a conversation in the little coffee shop at the edge of the main meeting space. She introduced herself as Arthur's wife.

Wait, what? Arthur's wife? Isn't Arthur married to Sally? I was smart enough not to say it out loud, but it took me a while to process the confusion. Then, as Russ and I drank our coffees, I watched the strange thruple share a snack at a table a few feet away. Sally was the Brookhaven wife; Priscila was the actual wife. I sat mesmerized as I watched Priscila handle the situation with remarkable class and dignity.

I wasn't sure if Russ would be interested in such a relationship since most of the female residents were so much older. In the beginning, he struggled with me not being there all the time. When I left, he got angry and caused a scene, and one of the managers had to intercede to calm him down. But after almost four months, he was accustomed to his new home. I often found him in the living room with Joseph and Daisy as they laughed and told jokes. They were an inseparable crew that moved from space to space, enjoying each other's company. I guess the relationship wasn't as platonic as I thought. My suspicions were confirmed by Holly's body language.

"I see. What's been going on?" I asked.

"Well, at night, he often ends up in her room. It seems to be becoming a thing. I don't think anything sexual is going on, but we wanted to let you know in case that changes."

"Wow. What's your policy on that?"

"When we see something, we separate them and notify the families, but that's about it as long as it's consensual."

I attempted to navigate the uncharted territory. "And what about Daisy's family? Are they okay with it?"

"Yes. Daisy likes companionship, so they weren't surprised that she sought someone here. They're fine."

I took a minute to process. "Well, if you all are okay with it, and Daisy's family is okay with it, then I'm okay with it. Seriously, I just want him to be happy."

"That's a great way to look at it. If anything changes, I'll let you know."

On my way out of her office, I turned and laughed. "I don't think I realized the intricacies of your job until now. Damn girl, life must get interesting."

She laughed back. "You have no idea."

That night after I put the kids to bed, I relaxed into my new reading nook, a little alcove on the side of my bedroom with a cozy chair and a rarely used fireplace. It used to have two chairs, but one of them went with Russ to Brookhaven, so I rearranged the furniture and decor to claim the space as my own. Instead of picking up my book, I sat back and thought.

Okay, Nicole. What do you honestly think about this? It was weird, but everything about my situation was weird. It was a dementia unit. Daisy wasn't a home hussie. She was a sweet, wonderful person who was someone's mom.

After I dropped off her Honey Bunches of Oats, Donna filled me in on the whole situation. "You know, she sits with us at meals. She talked about Russ, and I reminded her that he was married. She looked right at me and said that she knew that because he was married to *her*." Donna chuckled and went on, "Then I told her to stay the heck away from my husband."

Daisy probably did believe Russ was her husband, and despite all my time with Russ, I had no idea what he thought. Some days he seemed okay, and other days, he had no idea where he was. I couldn't begrudge either of them for the situation.

Dig deep, Nicole. What do you feel? I dug, and I realized that all I felt was relief. I prayed that Russ would find peace and dignity in the rest of his journey. What was better peace than the comfort of companionship? The man I married had left us long ago, and the man that now existed needed a presence I couldn't give. Daisy wasn't a threat; she was an enormous gift to both of us. The guilt barraging my conscience eased, and for the first time in a while, I felt free.

With Russ moving on in his life, I realized I also needed to move on in mine. The kids consumed a good chunk of my days, but the evening hours became mine. When Russ was home, if I went anywhere or did anything, he followed. So, for him to sit, I had to sit. The logical answer was to watch television. Now, as I watched TV by myself, I discovered that I hated TV. Countless hours staring at a box with nothing learned; it wasn't how I wanted to spend my time. I had a free license to do whatever I chose, whatever I wanted. I soon discovered I wanted to organize.

Months and months of Russ's disease reaped chaos throughout the house. He emptied the contents of file folders for sport. He hid trinkets in mysterious places to keep them safe. He disassembled tools and separated their parts to obscure the source. Night after night, I picked a project and brought order to the pandemonium. I mentally inventoried and found logical homes for each item, often heralded by the help of my new coveted label maker.

As the clutter cleared away, I moved to more significant projects I'd always wanted to tackle. My closet housed outfits I'd purchased decades ago and was ripe for a good cleaning. I culled and consolidated, but it still seemed cramped and messy. Then I walked out of my closet and stared at the two Scandinavian-style dressers in my bedroom. Since my closet was larger, Russ used both dressers for his clothes. They were his, even before we got married.

I couldn't use them, could I?

I walked by and straightened some towels in the bathroom, clearly delaying the decision that loomed. Soon, I was back, staring, almost paralyzed.

They're only dressers. Why are you making such a big deal of this?

They were only dressers, but they were *his* dressers. Some part of me still felt like he would come home and wonder where I put all his stuff, maybe even be angry. But the logical part of me knew that would never happen.

One by one, I emptied each dresser drawer and examined the contents. I found rarely worn clothes, old sweatshirts, out-of-style biking shorts, and scratchy T-shirts collected from a long completed shooting match. But there were a few finds that reminded me of who he was. There was the ridiculous Mao Tse Tung watch that he bought on his first trip to China. It had a regal image of the leader with his hand pulsing over the crowd, each wave announcing the passage of a new second. Russ laughed every time he ran across it and occasionally wore it to see how people reacted. Then there was his old tape recorder. Back when we first met, before iPhones and apps, he used the recorder to capture key meetings or random action items and thoughts. The tape still inside contained a recording of the two of us negotiating a licensing deal with the attorneys from a large electronics vendor. Most of it was mind-numbingly dull, but every few minutes, I heard him interject a clever point or ask a thoughtful question that reminded me of a different life. I packed items away in his closet, ready to move them but not to be rid of them.

I started with one dresser, then the other, and then the bathroom vanity. Once I finished the bedroom, I tackled the garage. Our neighbor, Rick Driscoll, was a great carpenter, and he helped me refurbish Russ's old workbench. Russ had taken a Dremel tool to the fiberboard to fix the tattered tabletop, leaving it a tangled mess of fluff. Now, Rick bolted on a new top, and Ryan helped me polyurethane it to make the bench like new again.

There were also two taxidermy masterpieces in the garage, Fred and Barney. Fred was a six-point deer that didn't qualify for trophy status. Russ had shot Fred while hunting on his own deep in the woods. As he collected his prize, a couple of serious rednecks pulled up on an ATV and claimed that they had shot the deer. The situation got heated as a huge black man walked up and weighed in. He claimed he saw the whole thing, and Russ was the one who shot the deer. The rednecks relented and drove off.

Russ struck up a conversation with his knight in shining camo and realized that he lived in the woods by himself. Too proud to take charity, the man offered to clean the animal if Russ gave him a little of the meat. Russ accepted and said that all he wanted was the tenderloin. Russ insisted, so the man agreed—but only if Russ shared his new batch of moonshine. They spent the entire afternoon drinking and telling stories while the man harvested the animal.

The event was so memorable, Russ made Fred a permanent wall fixture. His rack left much to be desired, so from then on, the rare times Russ went deer hunting, he took the antlers as a trophy. He then zip-tied these additions onto Fred, transforming him into a beautiful eighteen-point treasure. Russ called it "the antler club for men" with a giant glowing smile.

Barney was a scary-looking wild boar, the only one Russ ever killed. His fierce snarl was intimidating, but he often wore safety goggles or a Husqvarna helmet to make him more approachable. When we tried to sell Russ's house in New Hampshire, the fierce winter made the front door unusable. Snow covered the long walkway, and icicles on the roofline threatened to impale visitors with the slightest breeze. As a result, potential buyers used the garage as a means of entry. One day as we headed out to give prospective buyers privacy, a family of four walked in. A girl no older than five looked up at Barney with a look of pure horror on her face. When we got in the car, I looked over at Russ and laughed.

"There's no way in hell you're selling this house today. Barney went and screwed the whole deal."

I wasn't a dead-animal-on-the-wall kind of gal, but I couldn't get rid of Fred and Barney since they were now part of my misfit family. Instead, the kids and I decided to spruce them up a bit. Fred hung over our newly refurbished workbench. Hailey was in a massive unicorn phase, and we had several unicorn paintings that she and I had painted during girl time. A beautiful collage of rainbow unicorns complete with glitter and iridescent paint now surrounds our eighteen-pointer. I knew Russ would love our montage of *Larry the Cable Guy* meets *Queer Eye for the Straight Guy.*

Ryan, like every other nine-year-old boy, was into video games. His favorite game was *Jailbreak* on Roblox. One by one, the two of us painted the Jailbreak vehicles: the Mini, the Tesla, the Heli, the Ray, and more. Each one surrounded Barney and his bright orange safety helmet. Russ also loved fast cars, so I knew he would approve.

Project after project, I transformed the house until it felt like mine. So much of him was still there, but I selected the good and packed away the bad. I realized I *could* keep living in our house, a concept I was unsure of in the beginning. With spaces reclaimed and everything in order, I actually *wanted* to live in the house. It reminded me of Russ, and he was such a big part of me. I couldn't imagine letting it go.

Unfortunately, there were only so many closets and rooms to organize. The unknown for the next phase of my life started to plague me. I repeated the same questions over and over again. *Who am I? Who do I want to be?*

Throughout my career, I'd taken dozens of personality tests—Myers-Briggs, Gallup, DiSC—I had my reports, and they all brought a little slice of reality to my psyche. But the one test I spent the most time with was a lesser-known tool called ProScan. At its most basic level, it assessed four factors of behavior: Dominance, Extroversion, Pace, and Conformity. I'd taken the test four or five times, and every time, my result was the same. I was a "Midline" profile. I was a rare 2 percent of the population whose profile looked like a flat line heart attack when they mapped the four factors on their fancy chart, hugging the neutral axis right across the middle.

When I first saw this, I was surprised. Friends would describe me as outgoing, a leader, a driver. Surely these traits wouldn't lead to such a bland, flat line of personality? But as I learned more about the tool, I realized the roots of its results made perfect sense. I'd never scanned my parents, but if I did, I'd bet my dad was off the charts in Dominance and Extroversion. He was always the life of the party, and we couldn't get him *not* to voice his opinion, even if we begged. My mom, on the other hand, was high Pace and Conformity. She had infinite patience, went with the flow, and was a huge rule follower. I watched them growing up and noticed their strengths and weaknesses. I consciously tried to take the best from both of them and leave the flaws behind. So, as I stared at my result, it made sense. My brain melded their disparate personalities into a beautiful flat line.

My coach taught me that midline didn't equal banality; it symbolized adaptability. The further a trait was from the neutral axis, the harder it was to change or adjust. Being at the midline, I could dial my behavior up or down as the situation demanded. *Interesting.* After hearing this, I watched my interactions. Sure enough, it was true. When I worked with my team, I toned up my dominance and extroversion and became the leader they needed. Then in executive staff, I took a more passive role, listening, learning, and assimilating before I chose to speak up.

Armed with my new insight, I learned to exploit it. Before board meetings, I sought out my CEO and asked what he needed from me that day. He coached me accordingly.

"Today is more about the sales pipeline. You can listen and watch, and I'll let you know when to jump in." Alternatively, "Today, we need to sell them on our next generation, so I need you to show you are a rock star and that you've got it covered." *Yes, sir.* And I let it be so.

I also came to own that I liked being adaptable. It was probably the genesis of my love of start-ups. I threw myself into a young, budding company and became what they needed. Program manager? Sure.

I've got you covered. Marketing lead? Okay, show me what to do. Head of R&D? Yeah, pretty sure I can do that too. I combined my adaptability with my top Gallup themes of Learner, Achiever, Arranger, and Maximizer to dive in, learn the ropes, and figure out how to make it better.

But as I sat home in the quiet with the kids at school and no job to go to, I looked around. For the first time since I was nineteen years old, I didn't have a boyfriend or a husband as a constant companion. There was no flurry of activity from a job or school. I had no one to adapt to. It was only me. Well, me and two little humans who watched my every move.

Who am I? Who do I want to be? For the first time in my life, I wasn't sure.

I'd already fielded calls from colleagues offering opportunities. Some were for consulting, and some were for full-time gigs. As they described the fabulous little widget that promised to revolutionize medicine, the voice in my head that used to latch on and engage instead sat back and said, "Meh." I couldn't go back to the grind of someone else's vision. I wanted to create my own vision and start or join something that furthered it. The problem was, what the hell was my vision?

So, I started with the basics. Forget vision; I needed to get clear on values. What values were most important to me? I scribbled and erased and scribbled again, and after a few days, I came up with six core values that now grace the wall of my kitchen.

Number One: Health. I understand my body, mind, and spirit, and I prioritize the things that keep them strong. My journey showed me that without health, there was nothing else. It was the top, the pinnacle, the most important. And that didn't only mean exercising and eating right. They were essential, but it was also vital to listen to my body. I no longer accepted bloating or crankiness. I figured out what I ate that caused it and avoided that food. I recognized when I felt anxious or fearful, and I stopped and meditated to change my mindset. It wasn't okay to be out of shape, and it wasn't okay to be depressed. My body and mind were telling me something, and I needed to slow down and *listen*.

Number Two: Family. I embrace my family as my core, my rock, and my center. Those two little kids, my two crazy dogs, my parents, my brother—they were everything. In whatever I did next, I couldn't lose sight of that massive truth.

Number Three: Growth. I learn and experience every day and use the knowledge I gain as a beacon for others. Learning made me happy. It kept my brain healthy. My tragedy exposed me to fascinating advances in the microbiome, epigenetics, and metabolomics. These sciences would become the future of medicine once technology could harness and make sense of the information. I hungered to learn more, and I longed to bring that future to the present.

Number Four: Friends. I surround myself with amazing people, and I treat my good friends like family. Russ's disease was isolating. I craved the love and laughter of my friends. In my brief time back in the world, I'd reconnected with so many fabulous people. That tribe was a crucial part of keeping me whole.

Number Five: Independence. I cultivate the habits and routines that make me financially and emotionally independent. Russ and I had worked hard all of our lives. That hard work left me blessed with financial freedom and the opportunity to take time to heal. I realized that most people didn't live that way. My kids lived in a big house and didn't want for much. I needed to ensure they had the tools to grow independent. I wanted them to live within their means and be happy in the process. Happy—that part was critical. In typical midline style, I'd spent too much time letting the emotions of others dictate my mood, my feelings. I needed to take control and find happiness within.

Number Six: Fun. I seek fun and enjoyment in everything that I do. Russ had excelled at bringing joy into our lives. I'd always envied his humor and how he made everyone around him laugh. His disease surgically removed that from my house, and I wanted it back. I wanted my home to be a place to gather, a place of laughter, a place of warm memories.

So, there they were, the first-ever Bell Family Values. I didn't know where they would lead, but I knew if I held to them, I'd be proud of whatever laid ahead.

But while I strove to rebuild, Russ continued to decline. As he built a life at Brookhaven, my almost daily visits ramped down to about twice a week. I made sure that he showered and had the supplies he needed, we went for walks on a local hiking trail, or we'd go out for coffee and a haircut. It was simple and sometimes challenging, but I think it helped us both.

Then, in March of 2020, the COVID-19 pandemic hit in full force, and suddenly, everyone was in quarantine. Visiting access was shut down, and rightfully so. Our only interaction was through video conferencing, but he refused to sit still or engage most of the time. As time went on without any connection, he developed his own story of reality. He told staff members that it couldn't be me on the tablet because I was dead, a hurtful but understandable coping mechanism for a horrible situation.

Russ always hated showering with staff members' help, and without my regular interventions, his hygiene suffered. He refused care, sometimes violently. Almost exactly a year after Russ entered Brookhaven, his belligerence required treatment in a psychiatric facility. He needed his medications adjusted, and Brookhaven couldn't do that in an assisted living environment. I later found out that Russ suffered from a urinary tract infection and that inflammation had likely triggered his behavioral flares. After a month of treatment and medication adjustments, he was stable and returned to assisted living.

In my first video call with him after treatment, I barely recognized him. With no grooming services during the lockdown, his hair and beard were overgrown. His head and shoulders hunched over, making it difficult to make eye contact. His words were incoherent and muffled. Despite my time training in weird, mostly one-sided conversations, I struggled to connect or engage with him in any way. Friends asked if he recognized me, but I honestly couldn't tell. The lack of eye contact and jumbled words made it too difficult to decipher. I wasn't sure if it was the infection, the medications, or the stress of the whole situation, but the decline in one month was swift.

In the beginning, not seeing him because of COVID was hard. Eventually, if I was honest with myself, it felt like a backhanded gift. The pieces of him that once shimmered through were gone. Only a broken shell remained. Watching him lose control of his body and mind bit by bit was a torture he wanted to spare us. I couldn't spare him from it, but I know he didn't want the kids and me to watch firsthand. He wanted us to remember the man he was, and every day, I told the stories of that man to Ryan and Hailey.

22

A Walk in the Woods

July 2020

It was day 2,000,025 of COVID-19 quarantine. We just got back from visiting my parents in Florida, and as I put him to bed, Ryan planned the last week of his summer vacation.

"Mom, can we go to the lake tomorrow?"

The question caught me by surprise. "You mean the big beach near the boat launch? Tomorrow's Sunday, and if it's open, it will probably be crowded."

"No, Mom, not the big beach. I mean behind the house. We can walk the path by Mr. Graham's house. Can we go?"

It was a simple question. When Russ and I bought the house, it was what we wanted. Bring the kayaks, the fishing poles, the shotguns—infinite adventures right in our backyard. But Russ's disease stole the woods from us. It stripped away the comfort and connection. Now, the only emotion a walk through the woods brought was panic.

"I don't know, babe . . ." I started.

He cut me off, anticipating my answer. "Come on, Mom. We can cover ourselves in bug spray. We have an amazing lake in our backyard, and we never use it."

The look in his eyes was sincere. I wondered how much of my response was rational and how much was irrational. There were so many jumbled emotions that I couldn't see through the tangles.

"I know I'm crazy sometimes, but the fear is real to me. So much was taken from us." It felt like too much to share with a ten-year-old, but he'd lived it. He knew.

"Mom, I know how much it impacted us, but sometimes, you have to move on."

I paused, stunned by the wisdom in his words. It felt like a role reversal with him as the parent and me as the child. Maybe he was right. Maybe I was irrational, paranoid.

I relented. "Okay, maybe you, Tyson, and I can go down while the girls hang out at the Driscolls. We'll see what the day brings. If we do it, we'll have to *cover* ourselves in bug spray."

He beamed his gorgeous smile and settled down into the bed.

As I said my final good night and closed the door, I felt the familiar tightness in my chest. My private version of PTSD strengthened its grip, and my heart fluttered.

It's a walk in the woods. You did it with Russ hundreds of times before kids. Bug spray works. Use it and relax.

My inner voice tried to convince my inner fear. *A walk in the woods.*

The next morning was pretty typical. Early on in the pandemic, we decided to quarantine together with the Driscolls. The kids needed playmates, and I needed other adults to keep me sane. We settled into a simple summer routine: meet at 9:00 a.m. for a walk and develop a plan for the day. The boys decided to build a fall garden box at the Driscolls' house, and Rick headed to Home Depot to pick up supplies. Building the box would take all morning. I secretly hoped it would get me out of my tenuous promise to go to the lake. The girls came to our house, and the morning was quiet.

Right before noon, I heard Ryan come home. "Mom? Moooom?"

"I'm in my office," I shouted out.

I heard his feet clamor up the stairs. "Mom, what are you doing?"

"I'm catching up on a few things after being away. What's up?"

"Tyson is here too. I thought we could do lunch and then go down to the lake like we talked about."

I sighed. I should have known that my son's tenacity would never allow him to give up on what he wanted. It was time to face my fears. "Okay. Let's get everyone fed, and then we'll get ready."

All summer long, the kids preferred to hang out at our house, and since I wasn't working, I welcomed the extra playtime. I became a master short-order lunch cook, and all four kids were fed and happy in less than fifteen minutes. I whipped up a lettuce wrap for myself and watched Ryan and Tyson stare at me with anticipation. "Are you ready?" Ryan asked.

"In a minute. Let me finish, and then I need to change."

After we straightened up the mess, the girls took off for the Driscolls, and I went back to my bedroom to ponder clothing choices. I pulled out a pair of tan, lightweight pants I hadn't worn in years. Next, I chose a pair of hiking socks and pulled them up to my mid-calf, tucking my pants into the socks. It looked ridiculous, but I was beyond looks at this point. I put on my hiking boots. I used to wear out a pair a year when it was only Russ and me, but this pair was five years old and looked brand new. Finally, I selected a bright white T-shirt that made it easy to detect any unwanted stowaways.

Before we took off, there was the mandatory spray factory. I covered the three of us—boots, legs, arms, torso, hair, neck. When I finished, a plume of lemon and eucalyptus surrounded us like Pig-Pen from Charlie Brown. I wanted ticks in the next county to know we were coming.

As we entered the trail to the woods, Ryan looked over at me. "Are you okay?"

I took a deep breath. "I think so, but I hope you know how much I love you that I'm willing to do this."

He smiled, and we were off.

Over ten years had passed since I first walked that narrow trail. After Ryan was born, we went on hikes, but we stuck to official trails that were well kept. This trail was for neighborhood use, but since nobody had maintained it, it was overgrown with long grass that made my anxiety surge. But as I watched Ryan and Tyson forge ahead, my mind eased. Their excitement melded with our protective plume to give me confidence. Bit by bit, the beauty of the woods came back to me.

The path went along our neighbor's fence until it abutted the ranger trail that ran through the game lands. About a hundred yards down the ranger trail, we came to a small, shaded beach. The boys ran over and argued over how deep in the water they would go. They waded in carefully and eventually grew bolder, pulling further and further from shore. I gazed at the serene landscape. Most boats avoided the area since it was a shallow finger off the main lake. Russ and I had gone duck hunting there, and I knew it was full of beaver damns ready to entrap an unsuspecting propeller. The lack of traffic left the water smooth as glass, reflecting tufts of green everywhere the eye could see. I thought back to the first time I saw it with Russ. We reveled in wonder that such majesty was in our backyard. My mind drifted, and I pictured him fishing with Ryan and Hailey under a nearby tree. How wonderful that would have been. Every time I tried to fish, I caught only sticks. Another role he would have played that I didn't know how to fill.

The boys swam and played for about an hour, and then I motioned that it was time to go. I pulled my trusty bug spray out of my khaki pocket and reapplied the plume for their way out. After all, the water had washed it off.

I shook my head at how I'd been transformed. I first came to this lake as a carefree girl, deeply in love and ready to start a new life. Ten years later, I was a chronic worrier with embedded scars and angst. But I was still here, and I was still strong. Most importantly, I had a young family and a group of friends that filled the hole left in my heart. I was lucky.

As we walked home, instead of looking down at each blade of overgrown grass, I looked up. The sky was blue, and the woods once again brought me calm. One thought repeated in my head. *I love you, Russ, and I promise to make you proud.*

Epilogue

May 2021

When I first started writing these pages, all I could remember was the man Russ became. The true person he was seemed squashed out of my memory. Each neuron systematically rewired with a memory of pain, disappointment, or loss. But with each session of writing, reading, and rewriting, the good memories returned. Suddenly, a sly look from Ryan or a quip from Hailey reminded me of a story. Something that had seemed lost forever once again became real, and we laughed at the crazy antics of the man we loved.

I'm now the age Russ was when we first met. Late at night, I can't help but wonder what would happen if forty-four-year-old Russ met forty-four-year-old me. I imagine our adventures, our family, our lives. It would be fantastic. I know I can't bring him back, so instead, I channel him. Rather than rush into something, I step back and think. What would Russ do? What would he see that I missed? How would he add his humor? He can't be with me, but that doesn't mean he can't guide me.

Recently, I took the kids to Hilton Head, South Carolina, during their fall break. My parents met us there, and while they watched Hailey, Ryan and I biked almost every trail and beach on our side of the island. Russ had loved to bike, and riding around with a little mini version of him warmed my heart. One day, as we turned a corner, an alligator laid sunning himself at the edge of a pond. He was far enough away that we were safe, but Ryan was still a little unnerved.

Then suddenly, Ryan laughed, looked at me, and said, "You know what Dad would do? He'd look right at the alligator and say, 'Go ahead, try and get me. I could use a new pair of boots.'"

I laughed because I knew he was right. That's exactly what his dad would say, and the fact that he knew that made me proud.

Russ's journey continues. In March of 2021, COVID visitation restrictions were eased, and for the past few months, I've been able to see him. But Russ barely acknowledges my presence. He sits hunched over and communicates in mumbles. He is thin, frail, and seems like an entirely different person from the man I knew. Ryan and Hailey haven't seen their dad since pre-COVID, and I don't plan to take them. Russ wouldn't want me to.

I still live with the guilt that I couldn't save Russ. As I look back, I see I was probably foolish to think I ever could. I saw the signs too late. Doctors shuttled me out of their offices with useless prescriptions instead of finding a root cause. I put pieces together while the damage entrenched itself. He had not one but a complex compilation of serious issues where treatment and recovery were unclear.

I tell myself that it wasn't my fault. I did the best I could. Even the most advanced research labs can't save someone as far gone as Russ. But as those words repeat in my head, the only thing that echoes back is, *Bullshit!*

I refuse to accept that the best I can do is sit and watch as millions of people lose their identities piece by piece. Sure, I'll die eventually, but death by neurodegeneration is not a death I want for me, the people I love, or anyone for that matter. I lost the battle with Russ, but I want my story and my work to keep others from realizing that fate—to keep them healthy, self-sufficient, and strong. If I can do that, then all the pain and the loss will be worth it. What I learned along the way already helped Ryan become a happier, healthier, stronger, and more confident little boy. Someday, Russ will look down at us from heaven and take pride in that.

They say things happen for a reason. Frankly, again, I call, *Bullshit!* Lots of people suffer, and they are nothing but worse off because of it. What I believe in is a more active process. I have to *create* a reason for what happened. I have to be a beacon to help others, so they can avoid the traps that ensnared me. I have to use my background and skills to make it easier for patients and doctors to see the signs *before* it's too late and before the map is on fire. The *how* is still fuzzy, but the destination is clear. Going back to the way things were isn't an option. My journey has placed a calling on my heart that is too strong to ignore.

So, the time has come to release our story for anyone to read. As I unleash these inner thoughts, it occurs to me that I should feel vulnerable. I've always been a private person, and letting strangers inside the darkest times of my life should be scary.

But instead of feeling vulnerable or scared, I feel hopeful. I hope that someone reads this book and understands that it's a cautionary tale. I hope it empowers them to look past the stories they've been telling themselves and figure out the whys in the illness around them. I hope it encourages them to go beyond the litany of symptomatic diagnoses to find root causes. I hope it emboldens them to trust their gut even when doctors tell them there's nothing wrong or nothing they can do. I hope it pushes them to search for a doctor who listens and finds the right answers and the right treatments. I hope my story helps them get well, and get well soon. Because the sooner they start, the better. My story is what happens when it's too late, but their story—*your story*—doesn't have to be that way.

Acknowledgments

Living this book was life changing. I experienced deep trenches that I never want to see again. I realize that I wouldn't have made it out without help, without my tribe. I am grateful for you every day, and I look forward to our adventures ahead.

To Susan, Gene, Pauline, and Phil. Not having family nearby made this journey that much harder. You adopted our broken family and cared for us like we were your own. I couldn't have gotten through without your support. I am eternally grateful for all that you do for us.

To every friend who texted, called, and checked in on me— thank you. A special thanks to Kathy, Sarah, and Vicky, who came to visit when the insanity peaked. I had isolated myself in the unhealthiest way, and your presence helped keep me sane. Also, a thank you to Ashley. You epitomize the love and care of all nurses, and I'm proud to now call you my friend.

To Doug. Your snarky jokes and crazy stories helped keep Russ with us. I called you in some of the worst times because you knew not only Russ but also what it was like to care for him. Thank you for the support and the laughter that came along with it.

To Scott and Jodi. Thank you for opening my eyes and for being there every step of the way. Your encouragement made all the difference, and the promise of poolside martinis kept me moving on even the darkest of days. Keep the casita ready for us.

To Mom and Dad. Our morning chats are a treasured part of my day. I'm so grateful for the love and support you provided through this and throughout my life. I now understand the sacrifices required to be a parent, and I feel blessed for the opportunities and comfort that your hard work afforded me. I love you to the moon and back.

To Tiffany and Rick. You befriended us in our most desperate times. Most people would have raced for the hills, but you kept showing up, offering more help and more support with each visit. I honestly don't think I would have made it through this journey or COVID isolation without your help. Your family is my olive branch and my silver lining.

Writing this book pushed me well outside of my comfort zone—maybe two or three hundred miles beyond my comfort zone. But engineers love process, and Nancy Erickson, your process turned my scattered journal entries into a book. Your coaching and our Mastermind group were precisely the push and feedback I needed. Thanks to all of you.

To my Zumba partner, Kathy. Your early feedback and focus group helped me refine and improve the book, so I felt confident to release it to the world. Plus, your friendship, letters, and regular check-ins always bring a smile to my face.

Finally, to Ryan and Hailey. You are my everything. Watching you grow and learn is the spark that drives me every day. Never forget that your dad loved you and that you made him proud. Together, we will create our reasons.

About the Author

Nicole Bell is a medical device executive and entrepreneur with over twenty years of experience in developing and growth-stage companies. She is an engineer by training with degrees from MIT and Duke University in Materials Science and Engineering and Biomedical Engineering. She is also a proud mother of two children and two dogs and lives with her family near Raleigh, North Carolina.

Find Nicole on Instagram and Facebook @nicoledaniellebell

CPSIA information can be obtained
at www.ICGtesting.com
Printed in the USA
LVHW031115221021
701186LV00005B/128